Clinicians' Guides to Radionuclide Hybrid Imaging

PET/CT

Series Editors

Jamshed B. Bomanji
London, UK

Gopinath Gnanasegaran
London, UK

Stefano Fanti
Bologna, Italy

Homer A. Macapinlac
Houston, Texas, USA

More information about this series at http://www.springernature.com/series/13803

Thomas Wagner · Sandip Basu
Editors

PET/CT in Infection and Inflammation

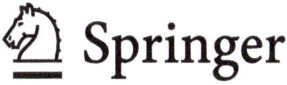

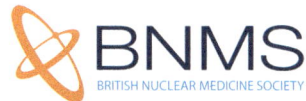

BRITISH NUCLEAR MEDICINE SOCIETY

Editors
Thomas Wagner
Department of Nuclear Medicine
Royal Free London NHS Foundation Trust
London
United Kingdom

Sandip Basu
Radiation Medicine Centre
Bhabha Atomic Research Centre
Tata Memorial Centre Annexe
Mumbai
India

Homi Bhabha National Institute
Mumbai
India

ISSN 2367-2439   ISSN 2367-2447   (electronic)
Clinicians' Guides to Radionuclide Hybrid Imaging - PET/CT
ISBN 978-3-319-90411-5   ISBN 978-3-319-90412-2   (eBook)
https://doi.org/10.1007/978-3-319-90412-2

Library of Congress Control Number: 2018947419

This Springer imprint is published by Springer Nature, under the registered company Springer International Publishing AG
The registered company address is: Gewerbestrasse 11, 6330 Cham, Switzerland

PET/CT series is dedicated to Prof Ignac Fogelman, Dr Muriel Buxton-Thomas and Prof Ajit K Padhy

Foreword

Clear and concise clinical indications for PET/CT in the management of the oncology and non-oncology patient are presented in this series of 15 separate booklets.

The impact on better staging, tailored management and specific treatment of the patient with cancer has been achieved with the advent of this multimodality imaging technology. Early and accurate diagnosis will always pay, and clear information can be gathered with PET/CT on treatment responses. Prognostic information is gathered and can further guide additional therapeutic options.

It is a fortunate coincidence that PET/CT was able to derive great benefit from radionuclide-labelled probes, which deliver good and often excellent target to non-target signals. Whilst labelled glucose remains the cornerstone for the clinical benefit achieved, a number of recent probes are definitely adding benefit. PET/CT is hence an evolving technology, extending its applications and indications. Significant advances in the instrumentation and data processing available have also contributed to this technology, which delivers high throughput and a wealth of data, with good patient tolerance and indeed patient and public acceptance. As an example, the role of PET/CT in the evaluation of cardiac disease is also covered, with an emphasis on labelled rubidium and labelled glucose studies.

The novel probes of labelled choline, labelled peptides, such as DOTATATE, and, most recently, labelled PSMA (prostate-specific membrane antigen) have gained rapid clinical utility and acceptance, as significant PET/CT tools for the management of neuroendocrine disease and prostate cancer patients, notwithstanding all the advances achieved with other imaging modalities, such as MRI. Hence, a chapter reviewing novel PET tracers forms part of this series.

The oncological community has recognised the value of PET/CT and has delivered advanced diagnostic criteria for some of the most important indications for PET/CT. This includes the recent Deauville criteria for the classification of PET/CT patients with lymphoma—similar criteria are expected to develop for other malignancies, such as head and neck cancer, melanoma and pelvic malignancies. For completion, a separate section covers the role of PET/CT in radiotherapy planning, discussing the indications for planning biological tumour volumes in relevant cancers.

These booklets offer simple, rapid and concise guidelines on the utility of PET/CT in a range of oncological indications. They also deliver a rapid aide-memoire on the merits and appropriate indications for PET/CT in oncology.

London, UK   Peter J. Ell, FMedSci, DR HC, AΩA

Preface

Hybrid imaging with PET/CT and SPECT/CT combines best of function and structure to provide accurate localisation, characterisation and diagnosis. There is extensive literature and evidence to support PET/CT, which has made significant impact in oncological imaging and management of patients with cancer. The evidence in favour of SPECT/CT especially in orthopaedic indications is evolving and increasing.

The *Clinicians' Guides to Radionuclide Hybrid Imaging* (PET/CT and SPECT/CT) pocketbook series is specifically aimed at our referring clinicians, nuclear medicine/radiology doctors, radiographers/technologists and nurses who are routinely working in nuclear medicine and participate in multidisciplinary meetings. This series is the joint work of many friends and professionals from different nations who share a common dream and vision towards promoting and supporting nuclear medicine as a useful and important imaging speciality.

We want to thank all those people who have contributed to this work as advisors, authors and reviewers, without whom the book would not have been possible. We want to thank our members from the BNMS (British Nuclear Medicine Society, UK) for their encouragement and support, and we are extremely grateful to Dr Brian Nielly, Charlotte Weston, the BNMS Education Committee and the BNMS council members for their enthusiasm and trust.

Finally, we wish to extend particular gratitude to the industry for their continuous supports towards education and training.

London, UK   Gopinath Gnanasegaran
                                                          Jamshed Bomanji

Acknowledgements

The series coordinators and editors would like to express sincere gratitude to the members of the British Nuclear Medicine Society, patients, teachers, colleagues, students, the industry and the BNMS Education Committee Members for their continued support and inspiration.

Andy Bradley
Brent Drake
Francis Sundram
James Ballinger
Parthiban Arumugam
Rizwan Syed
Sai Han
Vineet Prakash

Contents

Contributors

Ashik Amlani Department of Radiology, Guy's and St. Thomas' NHS Foundation Trust, London, UK

Alfred Ankrah Department of Nuclear Medicine, University of Pretoria and Steve Biko Academic Hospital, Pretoria, South Africa

Sandip Basu Radiation Medicine Centre, Bhabha Atomic Research Centre, Tata Memorial Centre Annexe, Mumbai, India

Homi Bhabha National Institute, Mumbai, India

Tehmina Bharucha University College London and Royal Free Hospital London, London, UK

Ashwini Kalshetty Radiation Medicine Centre, Bhabha Atomic Research Centre, Tata Memorial Centre Annexe, Mumbai, India

Homi Bhabha National Institute, Mumbai, India

Alok Pawaskar Radiation Medicine Centre, Bhabha Atomic Research Centre, Tata Memorial Centre Annexe, Mumbai, India

HCG Manavata Cancer Centre, Nashik, India

Deborah Pencharz Department of Nuclear Medicine, Brighton and Sussex University Hospitals NHS Trust, Royal Sussex County Hospital, Brighton, UK

Mike Sathekge Department of Nuclear Medicine, University of Pretoria and Steve Biko Academic Hospital, Pretoria, South Africa

Pradeep Thapa Radiation Medicine Centre, Bhabha Atomic Research Centre, Tata Memorial Centre Annexe, Mumbai, India

Thomas Wagner Department of Nuclear Medicine, Royal Free London NHS Foundation Trust, London, UK

The Role of FDG PET/CT in the Investigation of Pyrexia of Unknown Origin

1

Tehmina Bharucha, Thomas Wagner, and Deborah Pencharz

Contents

A critical appraisal of the role of FDG PET in Pyrexia of Unknown Origin (PUO) depends on an understanding of current concepts of PUO and systematic review of available evidence. This chapter provides an introduction to case definitions of PUO and summarises the current evidence, reviews available guidelines and discusses limitations in the application of FDG PET/CT for investigation of PUO.

T. Bharucha
University College London and Royal Free Hospital London, London, UK
e-mail: Tehmina.bharucha@nhs.net

T. Wagner (✉)
Department of Nuclear Medicine, Royal Free London NHS Foundation Trust, London, UK
e-mail: thomas.wagner@nhs.net

D. Pencharz
Department of Nuclear Medicine, Brighton and Sussex University Hospitals NHS Trust, Royal Sussex County Hospital, Brighton, UK
e-mail: Deborah.pencharz@bsuh.nhs.uk

© Springer International Publishing AG, part of Springer Nature 2018
T. Wagner, S. Basu (eds.), *PET/CT in Infection and Inflammation*,
Clinicians' Guides to Radionuclide Hybrid Imaging,
https://doi.org/10.1007/978-3-319-90412-2_1

1

1.1   Pyrexia of Unknown Origin

The origin of the term PUO is typically ascribed to Petersdorf and Beeson in their seminal work on 100 cases with 'a fever of >38 °c on several occasions for 3 weeks including 1 week inpatient investigation' [1]. Similar definitions are still used, essentially a protracted fever without a diagnosis after a reasonable set of investigations [2, 3]. Notably, the term is often used loosely and inappropriately to describe any undiagnosed fever.

There are a myriad of causes of PUOs, broadly categorised as (1) infectious, (2) inflammatory, (3) malignancy and (4) miscellaneous. These are elaborated in Table 1.1.

Table 1.1   Causes of Pyrexia of Unknown Origin (Adapted with permission [4])

Infections
– Tuberculosis
– Atypical presentations of pneumonia and urinary tract infections
– Vascular graft infections
– Intra-abdominal abscess, typically liver or diverticular
– Prostatitis
– Liver abscess
– Infective endocarditis or pericarditis
– Bone/joint infections ± infection of prosthesis
– Viral infections (EBV/CMV)
– Toxoplasma
– Imported/travel-related fevers that are not commonly seen (Brucellosis, Coxiella, Enteric fever, Yersinia, Bartonella, Leishmaniasis, Histoplasma, Blastomycosis, Coccidioidomycosis)
Inflammation
– Crystal arthropathy
– Polyarthritis (Rheumatoid arthritis, Seronegative Spondylarthropathy, Reactive arthritis)
– Adult-onset Still's disease
– Haemophagocytic lymphohistiocytosis
– Systemic lupus erythematosus
– Systemic vasculitis
– Thyroiditis
Malignancy
– Hodgkin's and non-Hodgkin's lymphoma
– Castleman's disease
– Renal cell carcinoma
– Hepatocellular carcinoma
– Acute myeloid leukaemia
– Hairy cell leukaemia
– Blast crisis of chronic myelogenous leukaemia
– Ovarian cancer
– Atrial myxoma
Miscellaneous
– Alcoholic hepatitis
– Drug-induced Fever
– Habitual hyperthermia
– Factitious fever

1.2   Rationale for FDG PET/CT in PUO

In spite of numerous attempts, there is no accepted investigational algorithm for PUO. Cases often undergo repeated, often discordant cycles of investigations including cultures, serology and imaging. Current estimates suggest that 20–50% of PUO cases remain undiagnosed, and there is a recognised associated mortality, particularly in the first few months [5–7]. Furthermore, there is a need to streamline the diagnosis to avoid unnecessary invasive investigations, exposure to reno-toxic contrast and radiation and to reduce costs. Some inflammatory causes of PUO are not associated with abnormalities in cross-sectional imaging or serological tests; while they may be steroid responsive, defining the diagnosis prior to presumptive treatment is useful for future management and to reduce unnecessary and invasive investigation.

Macrophages and neutrophils demonstrate high levels of the GLUT transporter [8]. Therefore, because FDG accumulates in areas of infection and inflammation, this could be useful in locating a focal source for the PUO. Additionally, the scans do not require the use of potentially nephrotoxic contrast, they also routinely scan from vertex or skull base to thighs, including parts of the anatomy particularly head and neck which are frequently not included in a diagnostic body CT.

1.3   The Evidence for FDG PET/CT in PUO

Since the introduction of FDG PET/CT, there have been numerous publications on the role of FDG PET/CT in PUO; however, there are more reviews discussing potential benefits than studies reporting evidence. A recent meta-analysis demonstrates the quality of existing studies is poor, comprising of retrospective case series of patients referred for a FDG PET/CT scan for the investigation of PUO [9]. The studies are largely confined to PUO in immunocompetent patients. The fact that the study populations are limited to PUOs referred at the discretion of the responsible clinician limits generalizability of conclusions about diagnostic yield. Overall diagnostic yield, the proportion of all FDG PET/CT scans (both normal and abnormal) that contribute to the diagnosis of PUO was reported as 56% (95%CI 50–61%); the heterogeneity statistic for the sub-group meta-analysis was $I2 = 61\%$ [9]. Importantly, only 5 of 18 included studies reported results of previous imaging, and a sub-group analysis estimated diagnostic yield beyond conventional CT is 32% (95%CI 22–44%), $I2 = 66\%$. The available evidence therefore suggests that FDG PET/CT scan may provide a finding that will help in making the diagnosis in approximately 32% of scans performed after conventional imaging has failed. There is currently no evidence to suggest which subsets of patients are more or less likely to have a diagnosis made with FDG PET/CT. An example of a contributive positive FDG PET/CT is provided in Fig. 1.1. FDG PET/CT helped to detect peritoneal tuberculosis in a patient with PUO.

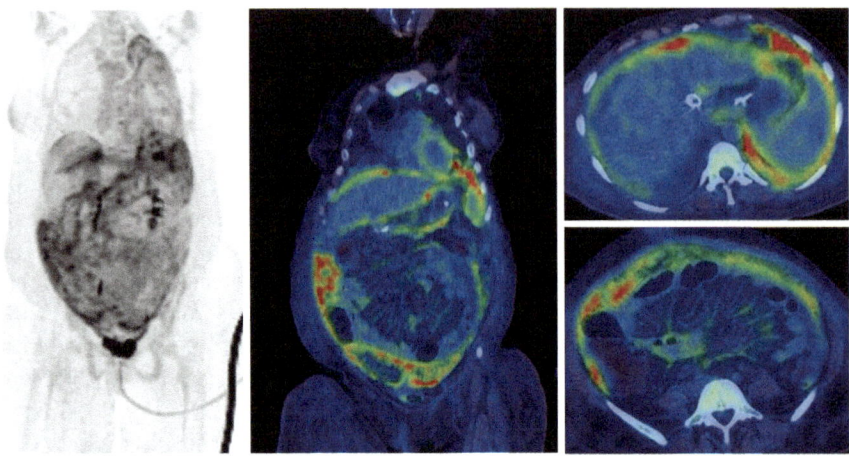

Fig. 1.1 A 41-year-old female with cryptogenic cirrhosis and portal hypertension, spiking temps despite amikacin/meropenem, blood cultures negative. CT shows free fluid, slight peritoneal enhancement. FDG PET/CT shows intense diffuse peritoneal uptake. Peritoneal biopsy is positive for TB

1.4 Limitations of FDG PET/CT in PUO

PET/CT will only detect some causes of PUO, e.g. some malignancies, foci of bacterial infections such as discitis and large vessel vasculitis. Other causes of PUO, e.g. drug-induced, non-routinely avid malignancies such as renal cell carcinoma, native valve endocarditis or many viral infections are typically not detected by PET/CT due to the inherent limitations of the technique. Negative scans do not rule out significant pathology. Additionally, the pattern of FDG uptake in the brain, heart, gastrointestinal and urinary tracts can limit the detection pathology in these regions. Accordingly, magnetic resonance imaging, transthoracic or transoesophageal echocardiogram, colonoscopy and urinary tract ultrasound may be more sensitive for pathology in these areas. Additionally, unless specially requested, the CT component is of lower quality than a diagnostic, higher radiation dose, contrast enhanced CT. Imaging post-PET may be needed for better definition.

1.5 Current Guidance and Investigational Algorithms

There have been numerous attempts to produce an investigational algorithm for the investigation of PUO; however, the geographical variation in cases and resources makes this a challenge. There are UK (Joint Royal Colleges) and European guidelines on the use of FDG PET/CT in PUO [10–12] which state that FDG PET/CT may be used after conventional imaging has failed to yield a diagnosis. A recent review on the use of FDG PET/CT in PUO also recommended using it in patients who have negative or equivocal findings at initial workup [13]. Some have advocated for early FDG PET/CT after a minimal set of investigations [3]. However, there is limited evidence that FDG PET/CT has a diagnostic yield over conventional imaging at the outset [9], and while use as a first-line investigation prior to conventional cross-sectional imaging is becoming more common, there is a risk of overuse in situations where specialist multidisciplinary clinical assessment and focussed investigations might be equally effective. We need better evidence that FDG PET/CT has a diagnostic yield over conventional imaging at the outset [9].

Conclusion

Identifying the cause of a PUO can be challenging and the theoretical advantages of FDG PET/CT are attractive. Although the quality of the evidence is weak, it has been shown to have diagnostic yields of 56%, and 32% over CT [9]. Current guidelines suggest using it when conventional investigations, including diagnostic CT, have failed to yield a diagnosis. However, the limitations should be kept in mind, and the understanding of the superiority of a tissue diagnosis retained.

Key Points

- FDG PET/CT is of value in patients with pyrexia of unknown origin and raised inflammatory markers. It can detect malignancy (e.g. lymphoma), inflammation (e.g. large vessel vasculitis) and infection. Its exact role, cost-effectiveness and the best time when to use it has not yet been validated by large studies.

References

1. Petersdorf RG, Beeson PB. Fever of unexplained origin: report on 100 cases. Medicine (Baltimore). 1961;40:1–30.
2. Knockaert DC, Vanderschueren S, Blockmans D. An evidence-based approach to fever of unknown origin. Arch Intern Med. 2003;163(16):1976–7.
3. Bleeker-Rovers CP, Vos FJ, de Kleijn EM, Mudde AH, Dofferhoff TS, Richter C, et al. A prospective multicenter study on fever of unknown origin: the yield of a structured diagnostic protocol. Medicine. 2007;86(1):26–38.
4. Bharucha T, Cockbain B, Brown M. Pyrexia of unknown origin: revisiting concepts to reflect on current clinical practice. Br J Hosp Med. 2016;77:579–83.
5. Mourad O, Palda V, Detsky AS. A comprehensive evidence-based approach to fever of unknown origin. Arch Intern Med. 2003;163(5):545–51.
6. Gaeta GB, Fusco FM, Nardiello S. Fever of unknown origin: a systematic review of the literature for 1995-2004. Nucl Med Commun. 2006;27(3):205–11.

7. Naito T, Mitsumoto F, Morita H, Mizooka M, Oono S, Ukimura A, et al. A multi-institution retrospective study on causative diseases and diagnostic methods for fevers of unknown origin in Japan: A project of the japanese society of general hospital medicine. J Gen Intern Med. 2013;28:S10.

8. Vaidyanathan S, Patel CN, Scarsbrook AF, Chowdhury FU. FDG PET/CT in infection and inflammation–current and emerging clinical applications. Clin Radiol. 2015;70(7):787–800.

9. Bharucha T, Rutherford A, Skeoch S, Alavi A, Brown M, Galloway J. Diagnostic yield of FDG-PET/CT in fever of unknown origin: a systematic review, meta-analysis and Delphi exercise. Clin Radiol. 2017;72:764–71.

10. Boellaard R, Delgado-Bolton R, Oyen WJG, Giammarile F, Tatsch K, Eschner W, et al. FDG PET/CT: EANM procedure guidelines for tumour imaging: version 2.0. Eur J Nucl Med Mol Imaging. 2015;42:328–54.

11. Buscombe J. Guidelines for the use of F-18-FDG in infection and inflammation: a new step in cooperation between the EANM and SNMMI. Eur J Nucl Med Mol Imaging. 2013;40(7):1120–1.

12. RCP/RCR/BSNM. Evidence-based indications for the use of PET-CT in the UK 2013; 2013.

13. Dibble EH, Yoo DC, Noto RB. Role of PET/CT in workup of fever without a source. Radiographics. 2016;36(4):1166–77.

PET/CT in Diagnosing and Evaluating Therapy in Vasculitis

2

Thomas Wagner

Contents

Vasculitides are defined by the presence of inflammatory leukocytes in vessel walls with reactive damage to mural structures. They are often categorised by the size of the vessels affected as large, medium and small vessel vasculitis. FDG PET/CT has shown to be an effective tool to investigate large vessel vasculitis. It is particularly useful because vasculitis can be difficult to diagnose given the absence of specific symptoms (e.g. fever, weight loss, malaise, fatigue, raised inflammatory markers). Morphological imaging shows anatomical changes and does not show inflammation in the early phase prior to structural changes. FDG PET/CT allows early detection of large vessel vasculitis before structural changes become detectable by conventional imaging. It is also difficult to distinguish active inflammatory lesions from residual anatomic changes due to previous inflammation [1, 2]. This book chapter will discuss the two most common causes of large vessel vasculitis, the criteria for

T. Wagner

Department of Nuclear Medicine, Royal Free London NHS Foundation Trust, London, UK
e-mail: thomas.wagner@nhs.net

© Springer International Publishing AG, part of Springer Nature 2018   7
T. Wagner, S. Basu (eds.), *PET/CT in Infection and Inflammation*,
Clinicians' Guides to Radionuclide Hybrid Imaging,
https://doi.org/10.1007/978-3-319-90412-2_2

PET positivity, differential diagnosis, the influence of immunosuppressive therapy, how PET can be used to change patient management, the evidence on PET for monitoring response to therapy, non-PET imaging used for the diagnosis of large vessel vasculitis and the role of FDG PET in medium and small vessel vasculitis.

2.1 Takayasu Arteritis

This rare disease mostly affects young women (80–90% of patients) with an age of onset of 10–40 years, with 1–3 new cases per million per year in the USA and Europe. Systemic symptoms include fatigue, weight loss and low grade fever. It primarily affects the aorta and its primary branches and subclavian artery involvement is common. A meta-analysis showed pooled diagnostic performance in estimating disease activity with sensitivity of 70.1% and specificity of 77.2%. FDG PET/CT compared to disease activity assessed by NIH criteria showed a sensitivity of 78% and specificity of 87%. The current literature is not clear on whether there is correlation between vascular uptake, disease activity and biological parameters [3–6]. Figure 2.1 is an example of a positive FDG PET/CT showing active large vessel vasculitis in a patient with Takayasu arteritis.

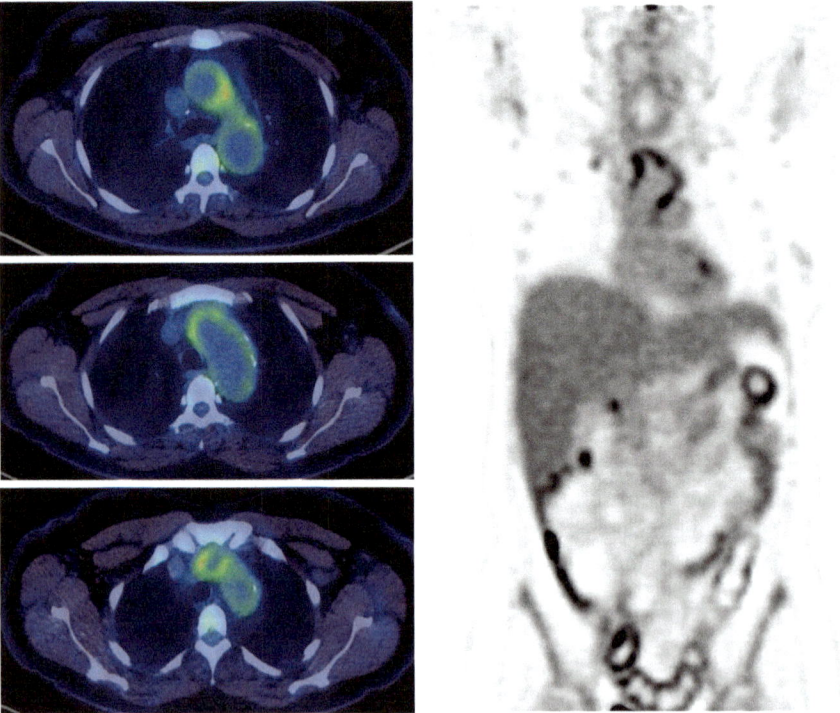

Fig. 2.1 Increased uptake in the aortic arch and the brachiocephalic trunk in a patient with Takayasu arteritis

2.2 Giant-Cell Arteritis

Mean age at diagnosis is 72 years. Prevalence is 1 in 500 adults >50 years. It affects predominantly the cranial branches of the arteries that originate from the aortic arch. Visual loss is a major complication. Temporal artery biopsy is the gold standard for diagnosis but has high false negative rates of 10–40%. There is a strong association with polymyalgia rheumatica. Pooled diagnostic performance for FDG PET is sensitivity 80%, specificity 89% and accuracy 84%. The main positive FDG vascular territories are the thoracic aorta, aortic arch, supra-aortic trunks and carotid arteries. There are discordant results for the correlation between vascular FDG uptake and serological markers (ESR, CRP) [7].

2.3 Criteria for PET Positivity

On visual analysis, a smooth linear or long segmental pattern of uptake in the aorta and its main branches with intensity higher than liver uptake is characteristic of giant-cell arteritis. A 4 point scale (0: no uptake, 1: uptake less than liver, 2: uptake equal to liver uptake and 3: uptake greater than liver uptake) showed that grade ≥2 for aorta and ≥1 for other arteries are positive for vasculitis [7–9].

Various teams have looked at semi-quantitative methods and compared uptake in vessel wall to blood pool, liver, lung and arterial uptake. The criterion that provided the optimal diagnostic performance was aortic arch SUVmax to venous blood pool SUVmax with a cut-off value of 1.53 that showed a sensitivity of 82% and specificity of 91% [10–14].

Figure 2.2 shows an example of diffuse smooth linear uptake in the wall of the aorta and its main branches, characteristic for large vessel vasculitis.

2.4 Differential Diagnosis

The main differential diagnosis of a positive PET for large vessel vasculitis is atherosclerosis, which can be quite difficult, especially in older patients in whom atherosclerosis is quite frequent. Typical findings for atherosclerosis are a patchwork of normal vessel wall, focal inflammation/uptake and calcifications. Typical findings for large vessel vasculitis are a smooth linear or long segmental pattern of uptake in the aorta and its main branches.

There have been anecdoctal reports of false positive findings with point spread function (PSF) reconstructions on the newer PET/CT cameras. The wall of large vessels is better delineated with PSF reconstructions and physiological uptake in the vessel wall is evident, which can make the vessel wall appear sharper and more intense. Careful attention to this finding is necessary when switching to a PSF reconstruction.

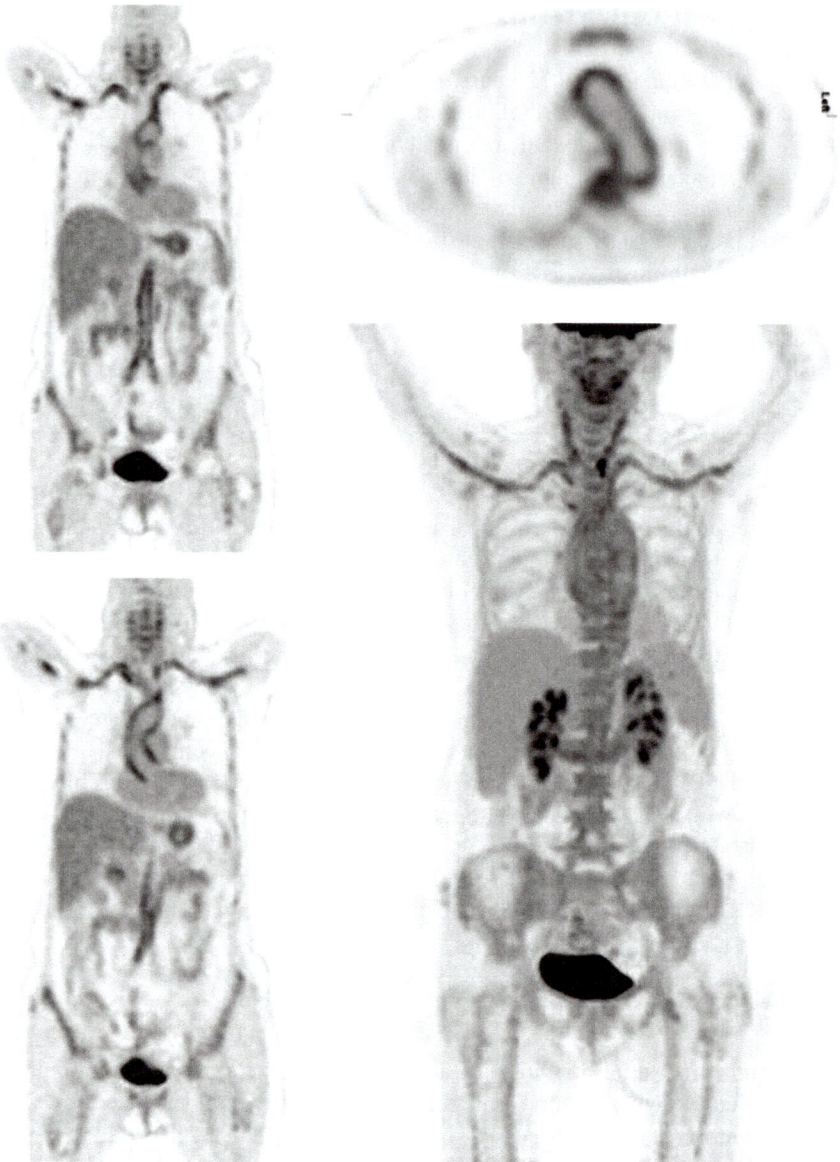

Fig. 2.2 Diffuse smooth linear uptake in the wall of the aorta and its main branches, characteristic for large vessel vasculitis

2.5   Impact of Immunosuppressive Therapy on Diagnostic Performance

The role of immunosuppressive therapy on the performance of FDG PET/CT was investigated in a study of 67 patients where a panel of experts determined the diagnosis and clinical management with and without the results of FDG PET. Large vessel vasculitis was confirmed in 30 patients and ruled out in 31. Six patients with inconclusive data were excluded. In the 30 patients not on immunosuppression, sensitivity was 99.6%, specificity 86% and diagnostic accuracy 93%. There was no false negative PET finding. In the 31 patients on immunosuppression, sensitivity was 53%, specificity 79% and diagnostic accuracy 65%. There were eight false negative PET findings [15].

2.6　Role of FDG on the Management of Patients

The same study [15] investigated how FDG results changed patient management. The addition of FDG PET results changed diagnosis in 28% of patients, leading to a reduction of the number of patients scored as indeterminate from 20 to 10. The diagnostic accuracy was 54% without FDG PET and 71% with FDG PET. FDG PET had higher additional diagnostic value in confirming than in ruling out large vessel vasculitis. There was no significant change in the number of indications for temporal artery biopsy. There was a change in the treatment recommendation in 25% of patients.

2.7　Role of FDG PET on Monitoring Response to Therapy

There is no good evidence showing that FDG PET has a role in monitoring response to therapy.

In one study 35 patients were scanned at diagnosis, on steroid treatment and at relapse. FDG PET was positive at diagnosis in 29/35 patients. FDG uptake in the wall of the affected vessels was reduced at 3 months of treatment but there was no further reduction at 6 months of treatment. The patients who relapsed had similar FDG reduction of uptake between the baseline and treatment PET than patients who did not relapse. The authors concluded that FDG PET performed in patients on treatment is not predictive of relapse [10].

Another study assessed FDG PET and MRI in 25 patients with complicated giant-cell arteritis despite immunosuppressive therapy. There was no significant correlation between PET findings, CRP and ESR and clinical findings. The authors concluded that MRI and PET were unreliable for assessing large vessel inflammation in patients with complicated GCA and pre-existing immunosuppressive therapy [16].

2.8　Morphological Imaging

PET and morphological imaging are complementary. FDG PET will show vessel wall inflammation before morphological changes occur. Structural imaging will show arterial wall abnormalities, occlusions and aneurysms that can persist after the inflammatory phase.

Colour-Doppler US can show a hypoechoic oedematous wall swelling (halo sign). Sensitivity is 75%, specificity 83% with temporal artery biopsy as gold standard.

High resolution MRI can show mural thickening, oedema, stenosis and dilatation. Sensitivity is 89% and specificity 75% using biopsy-proven disease as a reference. CT and CT angiography can measure aortic diameter in cases of dilatation and are useful in detecting mural calcifications and to assess concentric mural thickening [17, 18].

2.9   Medium and Small Vessel Vasculitis

Because of the limited spatial resolution of PET (4–6 mm) the involvement of medium and small vessels cannot be accurately displayed. FDG PET can sometimes detect vessel wall inflammation in medium vessels. FDG PET can detect organ involvement in small vessel vasculitis [19, 20].

Key Points

- FDG PET/CT is a sensitive and specific non-invasive test to assess patients with a suspicion of large vessel vasculitis. Its use is complementary to CT and MRI. FDG PET/CT should be performed before steroid treatment is started or within 3 days of starting treatment. It is not sensitive to pick up small and medium vessel vasculitis. Its role in assessing response to treatment is not clearly defined at present.

References

1. Treglia G, Mattoli MV, Leccisotti L, Ferraccioli G, Giordano A. Usefulness of whole-body fluorine-18-fluorodeoxyglucose positron emission tomography in patients with large-vessel vasculitis: a systematic review. Clin Rheumatol. 2011;30(10):1265–75 . Review. https://doi.org/10.1007/s10067-011-1828-9.
2. Cao Q, Chen W. FDG PET imaging of large-vessel vasculitis. PET Clin. 2012;7(2):227–32. https://doi.org/10.1016/j.cpet.2012.01.007.
3. Mavrogeni S, Dimitroulas T, Chatziioannou SN, Kitas G. The role of multimodality imaging in the evaluation of Takayasu arteritis. Semin Arthritis Rheum. 2013;42(4):401–12 . Review. https://doi.org/10.1016/j.semarthrit.2012.07.005.
4. Cheng Y, Lv N, Wang Z, Chen B, Dang A. 18-FDG-PET in assessing disease activity in Takayasu arteritis: a meta-analysis. Clin Exp Rheumatol. 2013;31(1 Suppl 75):S22–7. Epub 2013 Feb 25.
5. Arnaud L, Haroche J, Malek Z, Archambaud F, Gambotti L, Grimon G, Kas A, Costedoat-Chalumeau N, Cacoub P, Toledano D, Cluzel P, Piette JC, Amoura Z. Is (18) F-fluorodeoxyglucose positron emission tomography scanning a reliable way to assess disease activity in Takayasu arteritis? Arthritis Rheum. 2009;60(4):1193–200. https://doi.org/10.1002/art.24416.
6. Lee SG, Ryu JS, Kim HO, Oh JS, Kim YG, Lee CK, Yoo B. Evaluation of disease activity using F-18 FDG PET/CT in patients with Takayasu arteritis. Clin Nucl Med. 2009;34(11):749–52. https://doi.org/10.1097/RLU.0b013e3181b7db09.
7. Besson FL, Parienti JJ, Bienvenu B, Prior JO, Costo S, Bouvard G, Agostini D. Diagnostic performance of ^{18}F-fluorodeoxyglucose positron emission tomography in giant cell arteritis:

a systematic review and meta-analysis. Eur J Nucl Med Mol Imaging. 2011;38(9):1764–72. https://doi.org/10.1007/s00259-011-1830-0.

8. Meller J, Strutz F, Siefker U, Scheel A, Sahlmann CO, Lehmann K, Conrad M, Vosshenrich R. Early diagnosis and follow-up of aortitis with [(18)F]FDG PET and MRI. Eur J Nucl Med Mol Imaging. 2003;30(5):730–6.

9. Puppo C, Massollo M, Paparo F, Camellino D, Piccardo A, Shoushtari Zadeh Naseri M, Villavecchia G, Rollandi GA, Cimmino MA. Giant cell arteritis: a systematic review of the qualitative and semiquantitative methods to assess vasculitis with 18F-fluorodeoxyglucose positron emission tomography. Biomed Res Int. 2014;2014:574248. https://doi.org/10.1155/2014/574248. Epub 2014 Sep 1.

10. Blockmans D, de Ceuninck L, Vanderschueren S, Knockaert D, Mortelmans L, Bobbaers H. Repetitive 18F-fluorodeoxyglucose positron emission tomography in giant cell arteritis: a prospective study of 35 patients. Arthritis Rheum. 2006;55(1):131–7.

11. Lehmann P, Buchtala S, Achajew N, Haerle P, Ehrenstein B, Lighvani H, Fleck M, Marienhagen J. 18F-FDG PET as a diagnostic procedure in large vessel vasculitis-a controlled, blinded re-examination of routine PET scans. Clin Rheumatol. 2011;30(1):37–42. https://doi.org/10.1007/s10067-010-1598-9.

12. Besson FL, de Boysson H, Parienti JJ, Bouvard G, Bienvenu B, Agostini D. Towards an optimal semiquantitative approach in giant cell arteritis: an (18)F-FDG PET/CT case-control study. Eur J Nucl Med Mol Imaging. 2014;41(1):155–66. https://doi.org/10.1007/s00259-013-2545-1.

13. Moosig F, Czech N, Mehl C, Henze E, Zeuner RA, Kneba M, Schröder JO. Correlation between 18-fluorodeoxyglucose accumulation in large vessels and serological markers of inflammation in polymyalgia rheumatica: a quantitative PET study. Ann Rheum Dis. 2004 Jul;63(7):870–3.

14. Hautzel H, Sander O, Heinzel A, Schneider M, Müller HW. Assessment of large-vessel involvement in giant cell arteritis with 18F-FDG PET: introducing an ROC-analysis-based cutoff ratio. J Nucl Med. 2008;49(7):1107–13. https://doi.org/10.2967/jnumed.108.051920. Epub 2008 Jun 13

15. Fuchs M, Briel M, Daikeler T, Walker UA, Rasch H, Berg S, Ng QK, Raatz H, Jayne D, Kötter I, Blockmans D, Cid MC, Prieto-González S, Lamprecht P, Salvarani C, Karageorgaki Z, Watts R, Luqmani R, Müller-Brand J, Tyndall A, Walter MA. The impact of 18F-FDG PET on the management of patients with suspected large vessel vasculitis. Eur J Nucl Med Mol Imaging. 2012;39(2):344–53. https://doi.org/10.1007/s00259-011-1967-x. Epub 2011 Nov 10

16. Both M, Ahmadi-Simab K, Reuter M, Dourvos O, Fritzer E, Ullrich S, Gross WL, Heller M, Bähre M. MRI and FDG-PET in the assessment of inflammatory aortic arch syndrome in complicated courses of giant cell arteritis. Ann Rheum Dis. 2008;67(7):1030–3. https://doi.org/10.1136/ard.2007.082123. Epub 2008 Jan 26

17. Espígol-Frigolé G, Prieto-González S, Alba MA, Tavera-Bahillo I, García-Martínez A, Gilabert R, Hernández-Rodríguez J, Cid MC. Advances in the diagnosis of large vessel vasculitis. Rheum Dis Clin North Am. 2015;41(1):125–40, ix. Review. https://doi.org/10.1016/j.rdc.2014.10.001.

18. Pipitone N, Versari A, Hunder GG, Salvarani C. Role of imaging in the diagnosis of large and medium-sized vessel vasculitis. Rheum Dis Clin North Am. 2013;39(3):593–608. Review. https://doi.org/10.1016/j.rdc.2013.02.002.

19. Balink H, Bennink RJ, van Eck-Smit BL, Verberne HJ. The role of 18F-FDG PET/CT in large-vessel vasculitis: appropriateness of current classification criteria? Biomed Res Int. 2014;2014:687608. Review. https://doi.org/10.1155/2014/687608.

20. Soussan M, Abisror N, Abad S, Nunes H, Terrier B, Pop G, Eder V, Valeyre D, Sberro-Soussan R, Guillevin L, Dhote R, Fain O, Mekinian A. FDG-PET/CT in patients with ANCA-associated vasculitis: case-series and literature review. Autoimmun Rev. 2014;13(2):125–31. Review. https://doi.org/10.1016/j.autrev.2013.09.009.

PET/CT in Immunodeficiency Disorders

3

Alfred Ankrah and Mike Sathekge

Contents

Immunodeficiency disorders encompass a wide array of clinical conditions in which there is an aberration of one or more of the components of the immune system. These disorders may be primary or secondary to some other condition. Primary disorders usually become apparent in childhood but may present later in life. Secondary immunodeficiency disorders are more common [1, 2]. The last few decades have witnessed a steady increase in the population with immunodeficiency disorders. This is as a

A. Ankrah · M. Sathekge (✉)
Department of Nuclear Medicine, University of Pretoria and Steve Biko Academic Hospital, Pretoria, South Africa
e-mail: mike.sathekge@up.ac.za

© Springer International Publishing AG, part of Springer Nature 2018
T. Wagner, S. Basu (eds.), *PET/CT in Infection and Inflammation*,
Clinicians' Guides to Radionuclide Hybrid Imaging,
https://doi.org/10.1007/978-3-319-90412-2_3

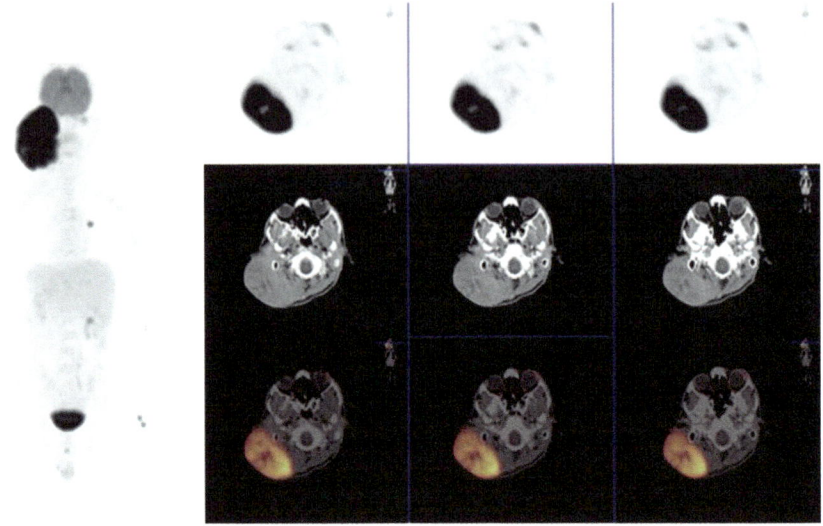

Fig. 3.1 A 36-year-old male with HIV infection with an undifferentiated sarcoma involving the right neck and a concurrent squamous cell carcinoma of the left eyelid. A metastatic lesion to the left lung is seen on the MIP

result of a number of factors. The high prevalence of HIV with 36.7 million infections worldwide is an important contributing factor [3]. In addition, advances in medical intervention have increased the immunocompromised population considerably. There are more patients in the posttransplant state who are on immunosuppressive therapy, more people using potent anti-cancer chemotherapy, and an increased survival of patients with hematologic disorders and malignancies [1]. Also, chronic disease such as diabetes mellitus and the use of drugs such as corticosteroids or immunosuppressant in inflammatory disease have added to the numbers. Finally, our increased understanding of underlying mechanism of immunosuppression with the discovery of new primary immunodeficiency has also contributed to this increase [1, 4].

Opportunistic infections occur in immunocompromised host over and above infections encountered by other people [5]. The clinical and radiological features of infections in the immunodeficiency state are usually diminished as a result of the blunted inflammatory response. This may delay the diagnosis. Malignancies on the other hand tend be more aggressive and occur in a younger age in certain immunodeficiency states [6, 7], see Fig. 3.1.

PET/CT combines functional imaging with anatomical imaging, and hence it is an important tool in the early diagnosis and management of conditions associated with immunodeficiency where anatomically changes may be diminished.

3.1   PET/CT in HIV

The clinical manifestation of patients with HIV is highly variable. Patients with HIV present with a wide range of infections, malignancies, and other disorders.

3.1.1   HIV-Associated Malignancy

HIV-associated malignancies are classified as AIDS-defining cancers (ADCs) and non-AIDS-defining cancers (NADCs). The ADCs include invasive cervical cancer, non-Hodgkin's lymphoma, and Kaposi's sarcoma. The rates of ADCs have declined considerably after the introduction of Highly active antiretroviral therapy (HAART); however, they are still elevated compared to the rates in patients without HIV. The NADCs include Hodgkin's lymphoma, lung cancer, hepatic and anal cancers; these cancers appear to have increased in the era of HAART [8–10]. The role of PET/CT in these cancers is similar to patients without immunosuppression and is outlined in Table 3.1 [11–13]. In cancers such as cervical cancer and aggressive lymphoma, FDG PET/CT is used in the initial evaluation before therapy, defining the extent of disease, predicting early treatment response, and assessing response at the end of therapy [15–18], see Fig. 3.2. FDG PET/CT may be used to distinguish primary CNS lymphoma and infectious space occupying lesions in the brain [19, 20]. In HIV-associated Kaposi sarcoma, FDG PET/CT is able to detect occult lesions which are difficult to detect on other imaging modalities [21, 22], see Fig. 3.3.

3.1.2   HIV-Associated Infections

TB usually manifests as a cavitatory lung disease frequently affecting the upper lobes. In the presence of immunosuppression such as HIV, the lesions tend to involve middle and lower lobes more often and cavitation occurs less frequently [22–24], see Fig. 3.4. Extrapulmonary TB is also more likely to be diagnosed in HIV [23, 24]. TB disease activity correlates with FDG uptake on PET/CT. FDG PET/CT can be used to detect TB, stage infection and assess response to therapy to TB [22–24]. In *Pneumocystis jiroveci* pneumonitis where there are differences in manifestation in different immunodeficiency disorders such as HIV and renal transplant recipients, FDG PET/CT has demonstrated its usefulness in early diagnosis [25, 26].

Table 3.1 FDG PET/CT in malignancies associated with immunodeficiency [12–14]

Diagnosis
- Determine site of biopsy
- Differentiation of benign from malignant lesions
- Carcinoma of unknown primary evaluation
- Detect sites of suspicious malignant lesions

Staging
Response evaluation
Restaging
Suspected recurrence
Follow-up
Radiotherapy planning
Prognosis—SUVmax, TLG, MTV

SUVmax maximum standard uptake value, *TLG* total lesion glycolysis, *MTV* metabolic tumor volume

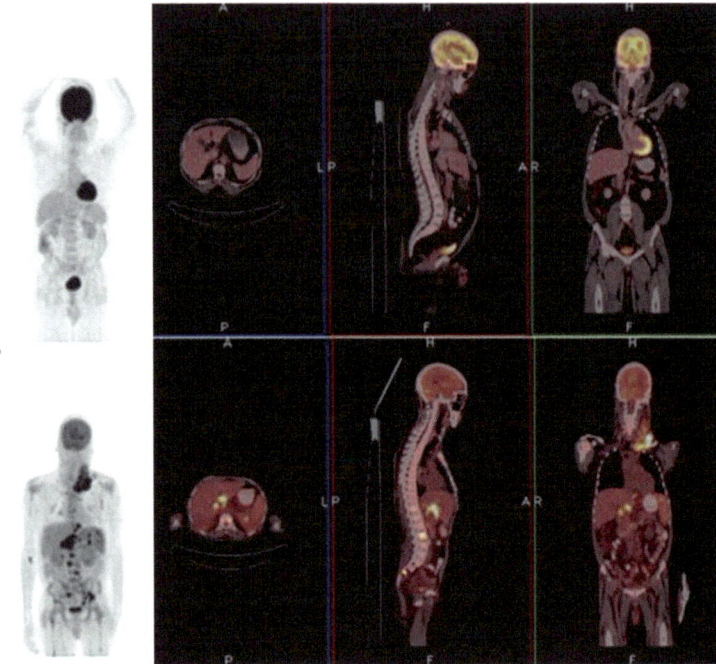

Fig. 3.2 Assessment of Hodgkin's lymphoma on completion of therapy. Top FDG PET/CT on completion of therapy. Bottom row baseline scan splenic, hepatic skeletal and nodes above and below the diaphragm. There is complete metabolic and morphologic response. Illustrates the use of FDG PET/CT at the end of therapy

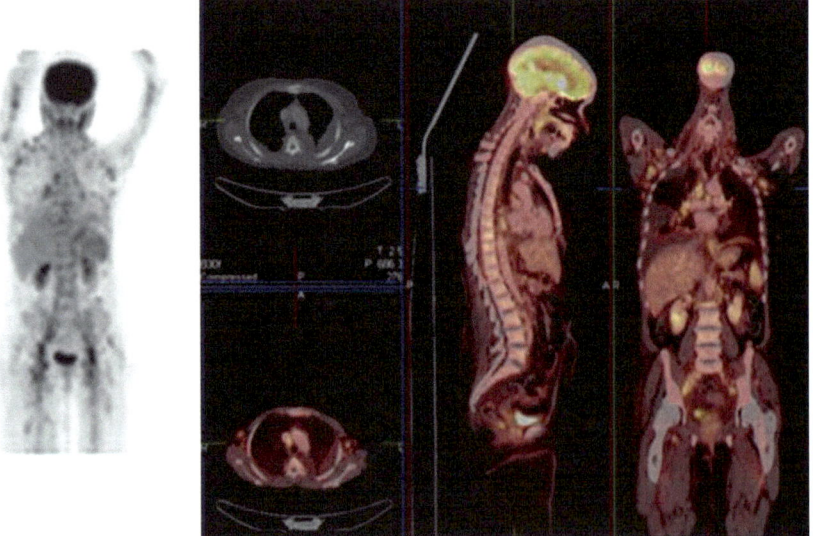

Fig. 3.3 Patient with HIV CD4 count 94 cells/mm^3 and viral load 1,158,944 copies per mL. Biopsy of the inguinal region revealed nodular Kaposi sarcoma. The axillary or mediastinal lymph also noted and may be related to HIV lymphadenopathy other causes of lymphadenopathy such as lymphoma or TB may only be excluded by histological assessment

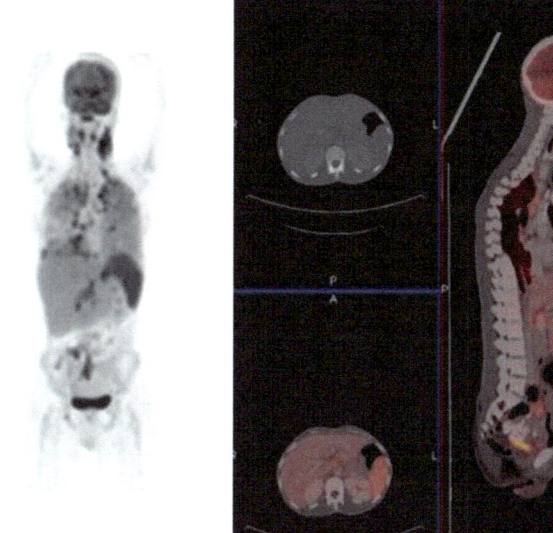
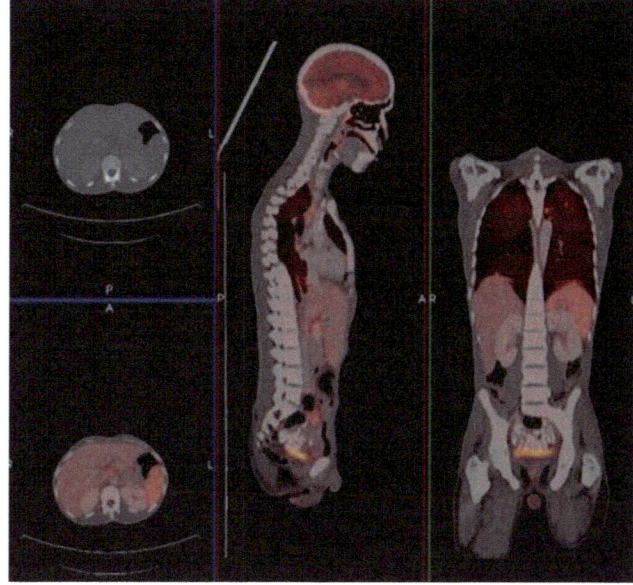

Fig. 3.4 HIV and TB coinfection demonstrating miliary TB of the lung and TB adenitis of the mediastinal and abdominal nodes. The spleen is much more intense than the liver. This demonstrates both atypical pulmonary and extrapulmonary TB encountered in the HIV patient

3.1.3   Fever of Unknown Origin (FUO)

PET/CT has been shown to be useful in evaluation of FUO [27, 28]. In HIV, viremia did not impede the performance of FDG PET/CT [29]. FDG PET/CT is indicated in HIV and other immunodeficiency states when initial clinical assessment and primary investigation do not reveal the cause of the fever [11].

3.1.4   Other Conditions in HIV

PET/CT has been shown to be useful in the management of conditions such as lipo-dystrophy associated with the use of HAART in HIV. These patients demonstrate marked increase of FDG in subcutaneous tissue which resolves when offending drug is withdrawn [30, 31]. Another condition where PET/CT potentially makes a difference is HIV-associated neurocognitive disorder (HAND). When dementia occurs in HIV, an increased subcortical uptake on FDG PET/CT scan after the exclusion of other causes of dementia is an early indicator of HAND [32, 33]. FDG PET/CT can detect carotid artery inflammation which may serve as an early marker to detect pro-artherosclerotic process in HIV patients who are at a higher risk of developing a stroke or myocardial infarction compared to the general population [34, 35]. FDG PET/CT has demonstrated that in well-controlled HIV patients with well-suppressed viral loads there is no increased arterial inflammation compared to people without HIV [36].

3.2   Transplantation

Patients undergoing solid organ transplant or hematopoietic stem cell transplant are at risk of developing secondary malignancies and infections due to the immunosuppressed state to prevent rejection [37, 38]. FDG PET/CT was found to diagnose these malignancies and infections with high sensitivity and specificity in solid organ transplants and hematopoietic stem cell transplant [39]. It is particularly specific for the detection of posttransplant lymphoproliferative disease [40]. FDG PET/CT may also play a role in the evaluation of gastrointestinal graft versus host disease [41, 42]. FDG PET/CT has been found to be a useful predictor of outcome of transplant in some lymphomas. There are however conflicting outcomes regarding the predictive value in pretransplant studies in non-Hodgkin's lymphoma [43–47].

3.3   Hematologic Malignancies

The role of FDG PET/CT in the various hematologic malignancies is considered in Table 3.2 [48–65].

3.4   Fungal Infections

Invasive aspergillosis and candidiasis and other invasive fungal infections (IFIs) are usually diagnosed in immunocompromised patient [66]. These usually occur in patients with hematological disorders, hematologic stem cell and solid organ transplant, intensive chemotherapy or primary immunodeficiency like chronic granulomatous disease [66, 67]. FDG PET/CT detects activity in different fungi and the

Table 3.2 FDG PET/CT in hematologic malignancies

Malignancy	Role of FGD PET/CT
Lymphoma	Staging and response assessment for aggressive lymphoma (Lugano classification) [48]
	Detects disease in normal sized nodes and more likely to determine splenic and diffuse bone marrow disease than other imaging modalities [49, 50]
	In early Hodgkin's and DLBC lymphoma may obviate the need for bone marrow assessment [51, 52]
	Detect and directs biopsy for transformation of indolent to aggressive lymphoma [53, 54]
Multiple myeloma	Characterizes osseous and extra osseous disease involvement [55–57]
	May replace routine bone marrow biopsy assessment during follow-up [58–60]
Plasmacytoma	Detects additional disease in patients suspected to have solitary plasmacytoma upstaging disease and changing management [61]
Leukemia	Not routinely used in management. In CLL may detect and direct biopsy when Richter's transformation is suspected [62–65]

FDG uptake corresponds to disease activity [67–69]. It was found to detect IFIs earlier compared to conventional imaging and to monitor disease activity and direct antifungal therapy [70–72].

3.5   Febrile Neutropenia

Febrile neutropenia (FN), a complication of patients undergoing myelosuppressive therapy is considered to be a sign of life-threatening infections. In FN however, infections usually lack localizing clinical signs. FGD PET/CT was found to be useful in detecting infectious foci including IFIs, septic emboli from central venous catheters. The high negative predictive value of FDG PET/CT facilitated the management of such patients [73, 74].

3.6   Inflammatory Conditions

Many inflammatory disorders use corticosteroid or other drug to depress the immune system in order to control symptoms of inflammatory disease. FDG PET/CT is able to monitor the activity of many of these inflammatory diseases and help determine whether the immunosuppressive therapy must be discontinued, increased, or maintained [75].

3.7   Diabetes Mellitus

Chronic conditions like diabetes are an important cause of immunosuppression. Conditions which frequently occur in diabetes where PET/CT can play a role are considered in Table 3.3 [76–84].

3.8   Limitations of PET/CT

FDG is a nonspecific tracer and the distinction between benign and malignant process becomes even more challenging in immunosuppression where granulomatous condition coexists.

Table 3.3 FDG PET/CT conditions frequently occurring in diabetes mellitus

Disorder	Usefulness of FDG PET/CT
Tuberculosis	Useful—Has been considered under HIV infections in this chapter [11, 22–24]
Osteomyelitis	Particularly useful in vertebral osteomyelitis [76]
Diabetic foot	Varying results have been reported [77–81]
Spondylodiscitis	Very useful [82]
Infective endocarditis	Patient preparation important and must be considered complimentary to other imaging modalities [83, 84]

3.9 Future Perspectives and Conclusion

Several other PET tracers are being used or are at various stages of development for management of immunodeficiency disorders. F18 Fluorothymidine (FLT) a marker of tumor proliferation whose uptake correlates with Ki67 and has been used in lymphomas. It is particularly useful for monitoring therapies containing cytostatic drugs [85–87]. Ga 68 CXCR4 targets the chemokine receptor expressed in many solid and malignant cancers. It is a potential therapy target for many cancers, especially hematologic malignancy [88–90]. Other tracers such as PET tracers could potentially have an impact on the management of immunodeficiency disorders [91]. PET/CT plays a major role in many immunodeficiency disorders. This role is likely to expand as new tracers are developed to deal with challenges faced in immunosuppressive disorders.

Key Points

- Immunodeficiency disorders encompass a wide array of clinical conditions in which there is an aberration of one or more of the components of the immune system. These disorders may be primary or secondary to some other condition.

- The clinical and radiological features of infections in the immunodeficiency state are usually diminished as a result of the blunted inflammatory response.

- Clinical manifestation of patients with HIV is highly variable. Patients with HIV present with a wide range of infections, malignancies, and other disorders.

- FDG PET/CT may be used to distinguish primary CNS lymphoma and infectious space occupying lesions in the brain.

- In HIV-associated Kaposi sarcoma, FDG PET/CT is able to detect occult lesions which are difficult to detect on other imaging modalities.

- TB usually manifests as a cavitatory lung disease frequently affecting the upper lobes. In the presence of immunosuppression such as HIV, the lesions tend to involve middle and lower lobes more often and cavitation occurs less frequently. Extrapulmonary TB is also more likely to be diagnosed in HIV.

- TB disease activity correlates with FDG uptake on PET/CT. FDG PET/CT can be used to detect TB, stage infection and assess response to therapy to TB.

- In *Pneumocystis jiroveci* pneumonitis where there are differences in manifestation in different immunodeficiency disorders such as HIV and renal transplant recipients, FDG PET/CT has demonstrated its usefulness in early diagnosis.

- PET/CT has been shown to be useful in the management of conditions such as lipodystrophy associated with the use of HAART in HIV. These patients demonstrate marked increase of FDG in subcutaneous tissue which resolves when offending drug is withdrawn.

- FDG PET/CT makes a difference in HIV-associated neurocognitive disorder (HAND). When dementia occurs in HIV, an increased subcortical uptake on FDG PET/CT scan after the exclusion of other causes of dementia is an early indicator of HAND.

- FDG PET/CT can detect carotid artery inflammation which may serve as an early marker to detect proartherosclerotic process in HIV patients who are at a higher risk of developing a stroke or myocardial infarction compared to the general population.

- FDG PET/CT has demonstrated that in well-controlled HIV patients with well-suppressed viral loads there is no increased arterial inflammation compared to people without HIV.

- Patients undergoing solid organ transplant or hematopoietic stem cell transplant are at risk of developing secondary malignancies and infections due to the immunosuppressed state to prevent rejection. FDG PET/CT was found to diagnose these with high sensitivity and specificity in solid organ transplants and hematopoietic stem cell transplant.

- FDG is a nonspecific tracer and the distinction between benign and malignant process becomes even more challenging in immunosuppression where granulomatous condition coexists.

References

1. Mortaz E, Tabarsi P, Mansouri D, Khosravi A, Garssen J, Velayati A, Adcock IM. Cancers related to immunodeficiencies: update and perspectives. Front Immunol. 2016;7:365. eCollection 2016.
2. Chinen J, Shearer WT. Secondary immunodeficiencies, including HIV infection. J Allergy Clin Immunol. 2010;125:S195–203.
3. UNAIDS. Global AIDS update 2016 UNAIDS report. http://www.who.int/hiv/pub/arv/global-aids-update-2016-pub/en/. Accessed 16 Nov 2016.
4. Verma N, Thaventhiran A, Gathmann B, ESID Registry Working Party, Thaventhiran J, Grimbacher B. Therapeutic management of primary immunodeficiency in older patients. Drugs Aging. 2013;30:503–12.
5. Fishman JA. Infections in immunocompromised hosts and organ transplant recipients: essentials. Liver Transpl. 2011;17:S34–7.
6. Bedimo R. Non-AIDS-defining malignancies among HIV-infected patients in the highly active antiretroviral therapy era. Curr HIV/AIDS Rep. 2008;5:140–9.
7. Kidd EA, Grigsby PW. Intratumoral metabolic heterogeneity of cervical cancer. Clin Cancer Res. 2008;14:5236–41.

8. Bonnet F, Chêne G. Evolving epidemiology of malignancies in HIV. Curr Opin Oncol. 2008;20:534–40.
9. Powles T, Robinson D, Stebbing J, et al. Highly active antiretroviral therapy and the incidence of non-AIDS-defining cancers in people with HIV infection. J Clin Oncol. 2008;27:884–90.
10. Shiels MS, Engels EA. Evolving epidemiology of HIV-associated malignancies. Curr Opin HIV AIDS. 2017;12(1):6–11.
11. Sathekge M, Maes A, Van de Wiele C. FDG-PET imaging in HIV infection and tuberculosis. Semin Nucl Med. 2013;43:349–66.
12. Poeppel TD, Krause BJ, Heusner TA, Boy C, Bockisch A, Antoch G. PET/CT for the staging and follow-up of patients with malignancies. Eur J Radiol. 2009;70:382–92.
13. Lee ST, Scott AM. The current role of PET/CT in radiotherapy planning. Curr Radiopharm. 2015;8:38–44.
14. Gallamini A, Zwarthoed C, Borra A. Positron emission tomography (PET) in oncology. Cancers (Basel). 2014;6:1821–89.
15. Herrera FG, Prior JO. The role of PET/CT in cervical cancer. Front Oncol. 2013;3:34.
16. Khiewvan B, Torigian DA, Emamzadehfard S, Paydary K, Salavati A, Houshmand S, et al. Update of the role of PET/CT and PET/MRI in the management of patients with cervical cancer. Hell J Nucl Med. 2016;19(3):254–68. https://doi.org/10.1967/s002449910409.
17. Gallamini A, Borra A. Role of PET in lymphoma. Curr Treat Options in Oncol. 2014;15:248–61.
18. Tateishi U. PET/CT in malignant lymphoma: basic information, clinical application, and proposal. Int J Hematol. 2013;98:398–405.
19. Heald A, Hoffman JM, Bartlett J, Waskin H. Differentiation of central nervous system lesions in AIDS patients using positron emission tomography (PET). Int J STD AIDS. 1996;7:337–46.
20. O'Doherty M, Barrington S, Campbell M, Lowe J, Bradbeer C. PET scanning and the human immunodeficiency virus-positive patient. J Nucl Med. 1997;38:1575–83.
21. van de Luijtgaarden A, van der Ven A, Leenders W, et al. Imaging of HIV-associated Kaposi sarcoma. F-18-FDG-PET/CT and In-111-bevacizumabscintigraphy. J AIDS. 2010;54:444–6.
22. Morooka M, Ito K, Kubota K, et al. Whole-body 18F-fluorodeoxyglucose positron emission tomography/computed tomography images before and after chemotherapy for Kaposi sarcoma and highly active antiretrovirus therapy. Jpn J Radiol. 2010;28:759–62.
23. Vorster M, Sathekge MM, Bomanji J. Advances in imaging of tuberculosis: the role of 18F-FDG PET and PET/CT. Curr Opin Pulm Med. 2014;20:287–93.
24. Ankrah AO, van der Werf TS, de Vries EF, Dierckx RA, Sathekge MM, Glaudemans AW. PET/CT imaging of mycobacterium tuberculosis infection. Clin Transl Imaging. 2016;4:131–44.
25. Skoura E, Zumla A, Bomanji J. Imaging in tuberculosis. Int J Infect Dis. 2015;32:87–93.
26. Ebner L, Walti LN, Rauch A, Furrer H, Cusini A, Meyer AM, Weiler S, et al. Clinical course, radiological manifestations, and outcome of pneumocystis jirovecii pneumonia in HIV patients and renal transplant recipients. PLoS One. 2016;11:e0164320.
27. Kono M, Yamashita H, Kubota K, Kano T, Mimori A. FDG PET imaging in pneumocystis pneumonia. Clin Nucl Med. 2015;40:679–81.
28. Bleeker-Rovers CP, van der Meer JW, Oyen WJ. Fever of unknown origin. Semin Nucl Med. 2009;39:81–7.
29. Keidar Z, Gurman-balbir A, Gaitini D, Israel O. Fever of unknown origin: the role of 18F-FDGPET/CT. J Nucl Med. 2008;49:1980–5.
30. Martin C, Castaigne C, Tondeur M, Flamen P, De Wit S. Role and interpretation of FDG-PET/CT in HIV patients with fever of unknown origin: a prospective study. J Int AIDS Soc. 2012;15(Suppl 4):18107.
31. Bleeker-Rovers C, van der Ven A, Zomer B, de Geus-Oei LF, Smits P, Corstens FH, et al. F-18-Fluorodexoyglucose positron emission tomography for visualization of lipodystrophy in HIV-infected patients. AIDS. 2004;18:2430–2.
32. Sathekge M, Maes A, Kgomo M, Stolz A, Ankrah A, Van de Wiele C. Evaluation of glucose uptake by skeletal muscle tissue and subcutaneous fat in HIV-infected patients with and without lipodystrophy using FDG-PET. Nucl Med Commun. 2010;31:311–4.

33. Rottenberg D, Sidtis J, Strother S, Schaper KA, Anderson JR, Nelson MJ, Price RW. Abnormal cerebral glucose metabolism in HIV-1 seropositive subjects with and without dementia. J Nucl Med. 1996;37:1133–41.
34. Sathekge M, McFarren A, Dadachova E. Role of nuclear medicine in neuroHIV: PET, SPECT, and beyond. Nucl Med Commun. 2014;35(8):792–6.
35. Yarasheski KE, Laciny E, Overton ET, Reeds DN, Harrod M, Baldwin S, Dávila-Román VG. 18FDG PET-CT imaging detects arterial inflammation and early atherosclerosis in HIV-infected adults with cardiovascular disease risk factors. J Inflamm (Lond). 2012;9:26.
36. Subramanian S, Tawakol A, Burdo TH, Abbara S, Wei J, Vijayakumar J, et al. Arterial inflammation in patients with HIV. JAMA. 2012;308:379–86.
37. Long B, Koyfman A. The emergency medicine approach to transplant complications. Am J Emerg Med. 2016;34:2200–8.
38. Katabathina VS, Menias CO, Tammisetti VS, Lubner MG, Kielar A, Shaaban A, et al. Malignancy after solid organ transplantation: comprehensive imaging review. Radiographics. 2016;36(5):1390–407.
39. Wareham NE, Lundgren JD, Da Cunha-Bang C, Gustafsson F, Iversen M, Johannesen HH, et al. The clinical utility of FDG PET/CT among solid organ transplant recipients suspected of malignancy or infection. Eur J Nucl Med Mol Imaging. 2017;44(3):421–31. https://doi.org/10.1007/s00259-016-3564-5.
40. Bianchi E, Pascual M, Nicod M, Delaloye AB, Duchosal MA. Clinical usefulness of FDG-PET/CT scan imaging in the management of posttransplant lymphoproliferative disease. Transplantation. 2008;85(5):707–12.
41. Bodet-Milin C, Lacombe M, Malard F, Lestang E, Cahu X, Chevallier P, et al. 18F-FDG PET/CT for the assessment of gastrointestinal GVHD: results of a pilot study. Bone Marrow Transplant. 2014;49(1):131–7.
42. Stelljes M, Hermann S, Albring J, Köhler G, Löffler M, Franzius C, et al. Clinical molecular imaging in intestinal graft-versus-host disease: mapping of disease activity, prediction, and monitoring of treatment efficiency by positron emission tomography. Blood. 2008;111:2909–18.
43. Johnston PB, Wiseman GA, Micallef IN. Positron emission tomography using F-18 fluorodeoxyglucose pre- and post-autologous stem cell transplant in non-Hodgkin's lymphoma. Bone Marrow Transplant. 2008;41:919–25.
44. Sucak GT, Özkurt ZN, Suyani E, Yaşar DG, Akdemir ÖÜ, Aki Z, et al. Early post-transplantation positron emission tomography in patients with Hodgkin lymphoma is an independent prognostic factor with an impact on overall survival. Ann Hematol. 2011;90:1329–36.
45. Sauter CS, Lechner L, Scordo M, Zheng J, Devlin SM, Fleming SE, et al. Pretransplantation fluorine-18-deoxyglucose—positron emission tomography scan lacks prognostic value in chemosensitive B cell non-hodgkin lymphoma patients undergoing nonmyeloablative allogeneic stem cell transplantation. Biol Blood Marrow Transplant. 2014;20:881–4.
46. Sauter CS, Matasar MJ, Meikle J, Schoder H, Ulaner GA, Migliacci JC, et al. Prognostic value of FDG-PET prior to autologous stem cell transplantation for relapsed and refractory diffuse large B-cell lymphoma. Blood. 2015;125:2579–81.
47. Gentzler RD, Evens AM, Rademaker AW, Weitner BB, Mittal BB, Dillehay GL, et al. F-18 FDG-PET predicts outcomes for patients receiving total lymphoid irradiation and autologous blood stem-cell transplantation for relapsed and refractory Hodgkin lymphoma. Br J Haematol. 2014;165(6):793–800.
48. Valls L, Badve C, Avril S, Herrmann K, Faulhaber P, O'Donnell J, Avril N. FDG-PET imaging in hematological malignancies. Blood Rev. 2016;30:317–31.
49. Schwenzer NF, Pfannenberg AC. PET/CT, MR, and PET/MR in lymphoma and melanoma. Semin Nucl Med. 2015;45:322–31.
50. Cheson BD, Fisher RI, Barrington SF, Cavalli F, Schwartz LH, Zucca E, et al. Recommendations for initial evaluation, staging, and response assessment of Hodgkin and non-Hodgkin lymphoma: the Lugano classification. J Clin Oncol. 2014;32:3059–68.

51. Adams HJ, de Klerk JM, Fijnheer R, Heggelman BG, Dubois SV, Nievelstein RA, et al. Bone marrow biopsy in diffuse large B-cell lymphoma: useful or redundant test? Acta Oncol. 2015;54:67–72.
52. Lim ST, Tao M, Cheung YB, Rajan S, Mann B. Can patients with early-stage diffuse large B-cell lymphoma be treated without bone marrow biopsy? Ann Oncol. 2005;16:215–8.
53. Noy A, Schoder H, Gonen M, Weissler M, Ertelt K, Cohler C, et al. The majority of transformed lymphomas have high standardized uptake values (SUVs) on positron emission tomography (PET) scanning similar to diffuse large B-cell lymphoma (DLBCL). Ann Oncol. 2009;20:508–51.
54. Barrington SF, Mikhaeel NG, Kostakoglu L, Meignan M, Hutchings M, Mueller SP, et al. Role of imaging in the staging and response assessment of lymphoma: consensus of the international conference on malignant lymphomas imaging working group. J Clin Oncol. 2014;32:3048–58.
55. Derlin T, Bannas P. Imaging of multiple myeloma: current concepts. World J Orthod. 2014;5:272–82.
56. Haznedar R, Aki SZ, Akdemir OU, Ozkurt ZN, Ceneli O, Yagci M, et al. Value of 18F-fluorodeoxyglucose uptake in positron emission tomography/computed tomography in predicting survival in multiple myeloma. Eur J Nucl Med Mol Imaging. 2011;38:1046–53.
57. Zamagni E, Patriarca F, Nanni C, Zannetti B, Englaro E, Pezzi A, et al. Prognostic relevance of 18-F FDG PET/CT in newly diagnosed multiple myeloma patients treated with up-front autologous transplantation. Blood. 2011;118:5989–95.
58. Sager S, Ergul N, Ciftci H, Cetin G, Guner SI, Cermik TF. The value of FDG PET/CT in the initial staging and bone marrow involvement of patients with multiple myeloma. Skelet Radiol. 2011;40(7):843.
59. Nanni C, Zamagni E, Celli M, Caroli P, Ambrosini V, Tacchetti P, et al. The value of 18F-FDG PET/CT after autologous stem cell transplantation (ASCT) in patients affected by multiple myeloma (MM): experience with 77 patients. Clin Nucl Med. 2013;38:e74–e7.
60. Usmani SZ, Mitchell A, Waheed S, Crowley J, Hoering A, Petty N, et al. Prognostic implications of serial 18-fluoro-deoxyglucose emission tomography in multiple myeloma treated with total therapy. Blood. 2013;121:1819–23.
61. Chargari C, Vennarini S, Servois V, Bonardel G, Lahutte M, Fourquet A, et al. Place of modern imaging modalities for solitary plasmacytoma: toward improved primary staging and treatment monitoring. Crit Rev Oncol Hematol. 2012;82:150–8.
62. Seam P, Juweid ME, Cheson BD. The role of FDG-PET scans in patients with lymphoma. Blood. 2007;110:3507–16.
63. Bruzzi JF, Macapinlac H, Tsimberidou AM, Truong MT, Keating MJ, Marom EM, et al. Detection of Richter's transformation of chronic lymphocytic leukemia by PET/CT. J Nucl Med. 2006;47:1267–73.
64. Rossi D. Richter's syndrome: novel and promising therapeutic alternatives. Best Pract Res Clin Haematol. 2016;29:30–9.
65. Stolzel F, Rollig C, Radke J, Mohr B, Platzbecker U, Bornhauser M, et al. 18F-FDG-PET/CT for detection of extramedullary acute myeloid leukemia. Haematologica. 2011;96:1552–6.
66. Kriengkauykiat J, Ito JI, Dadwal SS. Epidemiology and treatment approaches in management of invasive fungal infections. Clin Epidemiol. 2011;3:175–91.
67. Ankrah AO, Sathekge MM, Dierckx RA, Glaudemans AW. Imaging fungal infections in children. Clin Transl Imaging. 2016;4:57–72.
68. Ichiya Y, Kuwabara Y, Sasaki M, Yoshida T, Akashi Y, Murayama S, et al. FDG-PET in infectious lesions: the detection and assessment of lesion activity. Ann Nucl Med. 1996;10:185–91.
69. Hot A, Maunoury C, Poiree S, Lanternier F, Viard JP, Loulergue P, et al. Diagnostic contribution of positron emission tomography with [18F]fluorodeoxyglucose for invasive fungal infections. Clin Microbiol Infect. 2011;17(3):409–17.
70. Bleeker-Rovers CP, Warris A, Drenth JP, Corstens FH, Oyen WJ, Kullberg BJ. Diagnosis of Candida lung abscesses by 18F-fluorodeoxyglucose positron emission tomography. Clin Microbiol Infect. 2005;11:493–5.
71. Sharma P, Mukherjee A, Karunanithi S, Bal C, Kumar R. Potential role of 18F-FDG PET/CT in patients with fungal infections. AJR Am J Roentgenol. 2014;203:180–9.

72. Miyazaki Y, Nawa Y, Nakase K, Kohashi S, Kadohisa S, Hiraoka A, et al. FDG-PET can evaluate the treatment for fungal liver abscess much earlier than other imagings. Ann Hematol. 2011;90:1489–90.
73. Vos FJ, Donnelly JP, Oyen WJ, Kullberg BJ, Bleeker-Rovers CP, et al. 18F-FDG PET/CT for diagnosing infectious complications in patients with severe neutropenia after intensive chemotherapy for haematological malignancy or stem cell transplantation. Eur J Nucl Med Mol Imaging. 2012;39:120–8.
74. Vos FJ, Bleeker-Rovers CP, Oyen WJ. The use of FDG-PET/CT in patients with febrile neutropenia. Semin Nucl Med. 2013;43:340–8.
75. Glaudemans AW, de Vries EF, Galli F, Dierckx RA, Slart RH, Signore A. The use of F-FDG-PET/CT for diagnosis and treatment monitoring of inflammatory and infectious diseases. Clin Dev Immunol. 2013;2013:623036.
76. Palestro CJ. FDG-PET in musculoskeletal infections. Semin Nucl Med. 2013;43(5):367–76.
77. Familiari D, Glaudemans AW, Vitale V, Prosperi D, Bagni O, Lenza A, Cavallini M, et al. Can sequential 18F-FDG PET/CT replace WBC imaging in the diabetic foot? Nucl Med. 2011;52:1012–9.
78. Palestro CJ. 18F-FDG and diabetic foot infections: the verdict is…. J Nucl Med. 2011;52(7):1009–11.
79. Kagna O, Srour S, Melamed E, Militianu D, Keidar Z. FDG PET/CT imaging in the diagnosis of osteomyelitis in the diabetic foot. Eur J Nucl Med Mol Imaging. 2012;39:1545–50.
80. Gnanasegaran G, Vijayanathan S, Fogelman I. Diagnosis of infection in the diabetic foot using (18)F-FDG PET/CT: a sweet alternative? Eur J Nucl Med Mol Imaging. 2012;39:1525–7.
81. Nawaz A, Torigian DA, Siegelman ES, Basu S, Chryssikos T, Alavi A. Diagnostic performance of FDG-PET, MRI, and plain film radiography (PFR) for the diagnosis of osteomyelitis in the diabetic foot. Mol Imaging Biol. 2010;12(3):335–42.
82. Palestro CJ. Radionuclide imaging of musculoskeletal infection: a review. J Nucl Med. 2016;57:1406–12.
83. Gomes A, Glaudemans AW, Touw DJ, van Melle JP, Willems TP, Maass AH, et al. Diagnostic value of imaging in infective endocarditis: a systematic review. Lancet Infect Dis. 2016;17(1):e1–e14. https://doi.org/10.1016/S1473-3099(16)30141-4.
84. Gomes A, Slart RH, Sinha B, Glaudemans AW. 18F-FDG PET/CT in the diagnostic workup of infective endocarditis and related intracardiac prosthetic material: a clear message. J Nucl Med. 2016;57:1669–71.
85. Herrmann K, Buck AK, Schuster T, Rudelius M, Wester HJ, Graf N, et al. A pilot study to evaluate 3′-deoxy-3′-18F-fluorothymidine pet for initial and early response imaging in mantle cell lymphoma. J Nucl Med. 2011;52:1898–902.
86. Buck AK, Bommer M, Stilgenbauer S, Juweid M, Glatting G, Schirrmeister H, et al. Molecular imaging of proliferation in malignant lymphoma. Cancer Res. 2006;66:11055–106.
87. Hutchings M. Pre-transplant positron emission tomography/computed tomography (PET/CT) in relapsed Hodgkin lymphoma: time to shift gears for PET-positive patients? Leuk Lymphoma. 2011;52:15–1616.
88. Gourni E, Demmer O, Schottelius M, D'Alessandria C, Schulz S, Dijkgraaf I, et al. PET of CXCR4 expression by a (68)Ga-labeled highly specific targeted contrast agent. J Nucl Med. 2011;52:1803–10.
89. Wester HJ, Keller U, Schottelius M, Beer A, Philipp-Abbrederis K, Hoffmann F, et al. Disclosing the CXCR4 expression in lymphoproliferative diseases by targeted molecular imaging. Theranostics. 2015;5:618–30.
90. Philipp-Abbrederis K, Herrmann K, Knop S, Schottelius M, Eiber M, Luckerath K, et al. In vivo molecular imaging of chemokine receptor CXCR4 expression in patients with advanced multiple myeloma. EMBO Mol Med. 2015;7:477–87.
91. Vorster M, Maes A, Cv W, Sathekge M. Gallium-68 PET: a powerful generator-based alternative to infection and inflammation imaging. Semin Nucl Med. 2016;46(5):436–47.

PET/CT in Assessment of Sarcoidosis

4

Ashwini Kalshetty, Pradeep Thapa, and Sandip Basu

Contents

4.1   Introduction

Sarcoidosis is an intriguing multi-systemic disease of unknown aetiology. However, histologically it is characterized by cellular immune activity with formation of non-caseating granuloma in multiple organ systems [1], most frequently involving the lung. The challenge lies not only in diagnosing but also in

A. Kalshetty · S. Basu (✉)
Radiation Medicine Centre, Bhabha Atomic Research Centre, Tata Memorial Centre Annexe, Mumbai, India

Homi Bhabha National Institute, Mumbai, India

P. Thapa
Radiation Medicine Centre, Bhabha Atomic Research Centre, Tata Memorial Centre Annexe, Mumbai, India

© Springer International Publishing AG, part of Springer Nature 2018
T. Wagner, S. Basu (eds.), *PET/CT in Infection and Inflammation*,
Clinicians' Guides to Radionuclide Hybrid Imaging,
https://doi.org/10.1007/978-3-319-90412-2_4

subsequent management of patients owing to the non-specific symptoms, overlapping signs and diverse imaging features. Hence, it often remains a diagnosis of exclusion except when they present in acute stages, e.g. Lofgren's syndrome (triad of erythema nodosum, bilateral hilar lymphadenopathy and arthralgia). There are a number of clinico-biochemical-radiological pointers with imaging abnormalities can be detected on chest X-ray or HRCT but often poses a diagnostic challenge due to lack of sensitivity and specificity of the available tools. Hence, PET/CT has been studied extensively as an additional potential advanced imaging tool in the diagnostic armamentarium in the domain of sarcoidosis. This modality is of particular advantage in the following two aspects: (a) being a hybrid functional imaging tool with an ability to acquire whole body images, it is very useful for detecting not only thoracic disease but extra-thoracic sites as well with detection of occult sites that were previously unknown; extra-pulmonary sarcoidosis can be observed in 30–50% of patients with sarcoidosis (Fig. 4.1) and (b) it is already established that FDG PET/CT is extremely useful in assessing inflammatory activity and extent that would help in accurately mapping the

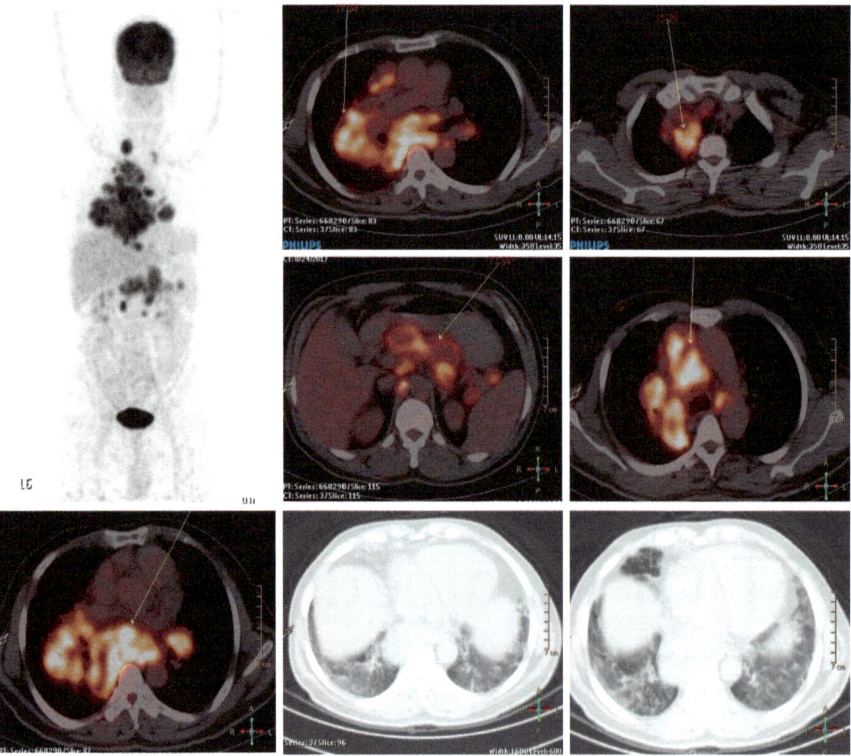

Fig. 4.1 A 43-year-old male, diagnosed with type II sarcoidosis. The biopsy from mediastinal nodes demonstrated chronic granulomatous inflammation. FDG PET/CT shows extensive disease in the chest and additionally uptake in the suprapancreatic and retro-peritoneal lymphadenopathy suggestive of extra-thoracic disease involvement

disease activity in a non-invasive manner. The latter application of FDG PET/CT has been extended to treatment response monitoring where it serves as an important sensitive and objective marker (Figs. 4.2 and 4.3). In this review, we have endeavoured to explore the various utilities PET/CT can offer in the course of sarcoidosis management.

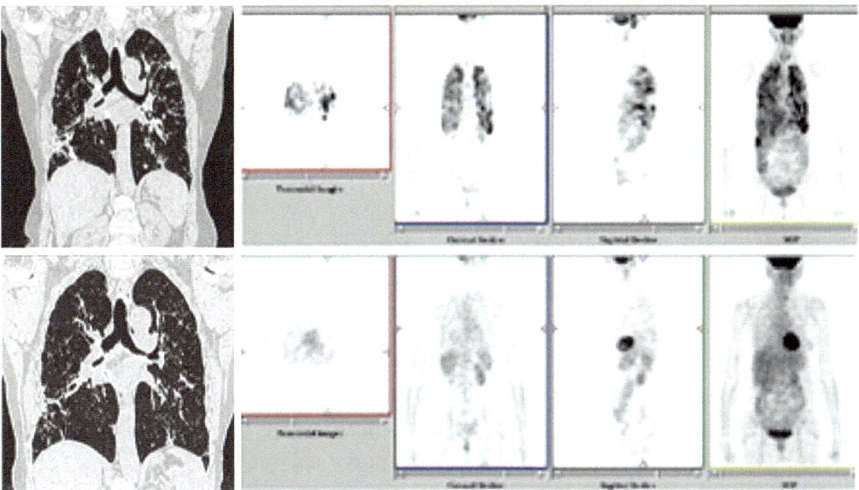

Fig. 4.2 FDG PET and HRCT in treatment response evaluation in pulmonary sarcoidosis (Reproduced with permission [55])

Pre-treatment

Post 6 weeks cortico-steroid therapy

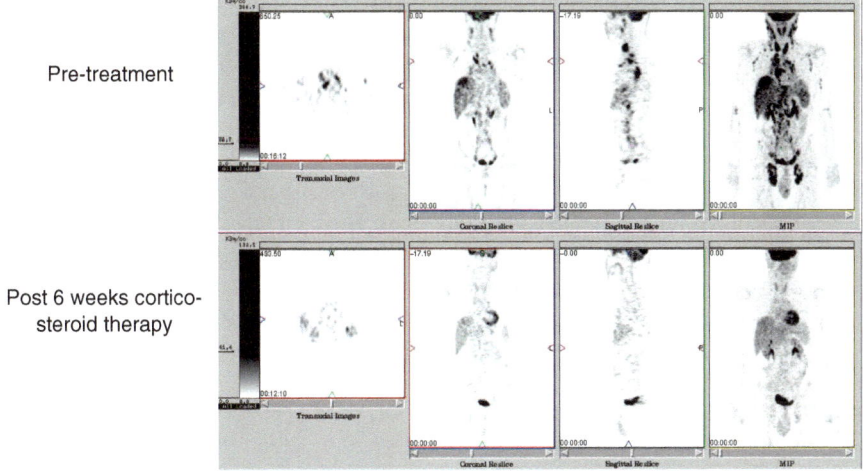

Fig. 4.3 Early documentation of therapeutic response at 6 weeks following corticosteroid therapy in patient with extensive sarcoidosis: promising role of FDG PET CT. The biopsy of the inguinal nodes was confirmatory of sarcoidosis. The uptake in bilateral thyroid gland is consistent with diagnosis of thyroiditis (which is frequently associated in this disorder) and the patient had history of hypothyroidism. This is predicted to be due to association of autoimmunity in this population (Reproduced with permission [56])

4.2   PET tracers

4.2.1 ^{18}F-Fluorodeoxyglucose PET/CT

^{18}F-FDG is the most commonly used PET tracer worldwide, bulk of the indication being oncology, however due to high uptake in inflammatory cells, it is also the most common tracer utilized in the evaluation of sarcoidosis. The hybrid modality combining both metabolic (PET) and anatomical imaging (CT) has enabled accurate localization and attenuation correction with possibility of studying both metabolic and morphological changes in the same imaging study. Traditionally, Ga-67 had been extensively used for the imaging of sarcoidosis but various studies have shown more accurate assessment of extent of disease involvement with ^{18}F-FDG PET/CT, including its ability of quantification of disease status [2–4]. The earliest demonstration of FDG accumulation was reported by Lewis et al. in both thoracic and extra-thoracic sites [5]. The sensitivity of ^{18}F-FDG PET has been reported 100% for pulmonary sites and 90% for extra-pulmonary sites by Nishiyama et al. [4]. Due to non-specificity of FDG PET/CT, it is not the modality of choice for diagnosis or screening purposes, however, can be utilized after the routine investigations fail to provide adequate diagnosis. FDG PET/CT certainly helps in uncovering the occult sites, as demonstrated in two large cohort studies how PET has certainly helped in uncovering new occult sites of active disease previously unknown [6, 7].

Diagnostic yield compared with serological markers
Around 60% of patients demonstrate high serum angiotensin-converting enzyme (ACE) levels though the serum ACE levels do not always correlate well with severity or extent of disease and in treatment response assessment. In a retrospective study of 36 proven cases of sarcoidosis, by Keijsers et al., ^{18}FDG PET was found positive in 94% of patients. In the same population, angiotensin-converting enzyme (ACE) and soluble interleukin-2 receptor (sIL-2R), the serological markers were positive in 36% and 47%, respectively [8]. Hence, FDG PET/CT can be useful as a baseline test to document active sites of sarcoidosis in patients with strong clinical suspicion but negative serological markers. Most patients present with non-specific constitutional symptoms rather than organ-specific symptoms. Hence, FDG PET/CT imaging may serve as a non-invasive tool to narrow down differentials and also to increase the yield of biopsy. We must mention here that the FDG uptake can mimic the lymph node involvement by malignancy, hence histological confirmation is mandatory.

4.2.2   Other PET Tracers Utilized in Sarcoidosis

4.2.2.1 ^{68}Ga-DOTATATE PET/CT
It is known that somatostatin receptor is over-expressed in inflammatory cells, especially activated macrophages [9]. The in vitro autoradiography of histological biopsies of sarcoidosis has shown that epithelioid cells and giant cells

expressed abundance of somatostatin receptor type 2 [10]. ^{68}Ga-DOTATATE has high affinity for somatostatin receptor(SSTR) subtype 2 and 5 and hence soma-tostatin receptor imaging (SSRI) is sometimes useful in inflammatory condition. In a study by Soydal et al., 8 previously diagnosed patients were evaluated with ^{68}Ga-DOTATATE, 5 patients with active disease demonstrated various degree of tracer accumulation while in 3 patients with chronic inactive disease, the study was normal [11].

4.2.2.2 ^{68}Ga-DOTATOC PET/CT
In another study by Nobashi et al., comparative evaluation of (68)Ga-DOTATOC PET/CT ^{67}Ga-scintigraphy (GS) in 20 patients of sarcoidosis documented ^{68}Ga-DOTATOC-PET/CT positive in 19 patients and negative in one patient with chronic inactive sarcoidosis, whereas GS was positive in 17 patients [12]. The inves-tigators concluded PET/CT with ^{68}Ga-DOTATOC may be superior to conventional gallium-67 scintigraphy in detecting sarcoidosis lesions, especially in lymph nodes, uvea, and muscles.

4.2.2.3 Experimental PET tracers
In a study by Kim SK, et al. for a patient with myelopathic symptoms and signs, patient was evaluated with multiple investigations including F-18 FDG and F-18 FLT PET/CT, with definite diagnosis by histopathology. They opined that F-18 FDG-avid lymphadenopathies with mild ^{18}F-FLT uptake can be characteristic find-ing of sarcoidosis and the combination of ^{18}F-FDG and ^{18}F-FLT PET/CT can be helpful in differentiating granulomatous inflammatory diseases such as neurosar-coidosis from malignancy.

Yamada et al. evaluated the FDG/Met uptake ratio using ^{18}F-FDG and 11C-Methionine PET to reflect differential granulomatous status in sarcoidosis and whether it can be a useful tool for pre-treatment evaluation. They could divide patients into the FDG-dominant group (FDG/Met uptake ratio $\geq$ 2) and the Met-dominant group (FDG/Met uptake ratio < 2) and the study show the rate of improve-ment assessed by clinical status and chest radiographs was considerably higher in the FDG (78%) than in the Met-dominant group (33%).

4.3   Initial Diagnosis

Due to non-specific symptoms and sign and diverse imaging characteristics, accu-rate evaluation of pulmonary and/or extra-pulmonary organ involvement of sarcoid-osis remains one of the great challenges and includes the assessment of sarcoidosis activity in a specific organ and its functional consequences [13]. Since whole body imaging is possible with FDG PET, in the past decade or so PET with ^{18}F-FDG, has emerged as a potentially powerful tool to visualize the intensity and extent of inflammatory activity of sarcoidosis throughout the body [2, 6, 8] and also helping in guiding the potential sites of biopsy.

4.3.1 Pulmonary Sarcoidosis

Lungs are commonly involved in sarcoidosis (>90%). Most of them resolve spontaneously but about one third of the patients progress to fibrosis causing debilitating symptoms. Chest X-ray (CXR) is the most commonly used imaging modality and the Scadding staging system based on X-rays is very useful from prognostication point of view (as patient with lower CXR more likely experience resolution of CXR abnormalities), but doesn't definitively decide initiation of therapy [14, 15]. Broncho-alveolar lavage (BAL) fluid analysis demonstrates characteristically increased CD3/CD4 lymphocytosis in active sarcoidosis and HRCT correlates with respiratory function impairment in sarcoidosis [16, 17]. FDG PET/CT may show diffuse or multi-focal uptake pattern, but the severity of pulmonary involvement as assessed by HRCT features and lung function parameters correlated with the PET activity in sarcoidosis [18]. Brudin et al. demonstrated that regional glucose metabolism in pulmonary disease is related to severity [19]. So total glucose hypermetabolism may be related to extent and activity of disease. The extent of disease activity may correlate with pulmonary function. Diffuse uptake in lung parenchyma which are left untreated suggest poor prognosis. Metabolic activity helps in choosing patients to initiate therapy or for observation. There is a linear relationship of diffuse FDG uptake with change in pulmonary function tests post-treatment [20] and one study also demonstrated that FDG uptake was related to ACE levels [21].

4.3.2 Extra-Pulmonary Sarcoidosis

4.3.2.1 Lymphadenopathy

Most commonly involved group of lymph nodes in sarcoidosis is mediastinal and hilar lymph nodes but enlarged lymph nodes are not exclusive of sarcoidosis as several conditions like tuberculosis or malignancy can present with lymphadenopathy. Various studies have utilized parameter like standardized uptake value (SUV) for categorizing lymph nodes as benign and malignant, even with dual tracer-like FDG and FLT [22, 23]; however, no significant differences were identified. Mediastinoscopy is done for histological examination and disease confirmation.

4.3.2.2 Cardiac

Cardiac involvement occurs in up to 25% of patients based on autopsy studies [24, 25]. Around 5% of patient manifest clinically with non-specific sign and symptoms, presenting with conduction disorders, congestive heart failure or sudden cardiac death and carries high risk of mortality and morbidity, accounting for 13–25% of fatal cases [26, 27]. The clinical diagnosis of cardiac sarcoidosis had been customarily established based on the Japanese Ministry of Health and Welfare Diagnostic

Table 4.1 Cardiac sarcoidosis evaluation with FDG PET/CT: original studies and systematic review

Author (year)/study type	No of patients	PET tracer	Sensitivity and specificity
Ohira (2007)/prospective	21	FDG	88 and 39%
Yamagashi (2003)/ prospective	17	FDG, NH3	FDG uptake (82% sensitivity) NH3 defect (76% sensitivity)
Tahara (2010)/prospective	24	FDG	100 and 97%
Youssef (2012)/systematic review	164	FDG	89 and 78%

Guidelines (JMHW) [28]. This was later revised by the Japan Society of Sarcoidosis and other Granulomatous Disorders in 2006 [29]. Some of the studies using PET tracers for diagnosis of cardiac sarcopidosis are summarized below (Table 4.1).

Various studies have evaluated the value of cardiac ^{18}F-FDG PET imaging for assessment of active cardiac sarcoidosis and now is being routinely undertaken for the many centres [30–32]. The criteria for clinical diagnosis of cardiac sarcoidosis that includes PET imaging has been established by Heart Rhythm Society [33]. It appears that the combined use of FDG PET/CT and cardiac MR would provide the best results in cardiac sarcoidosis that could allow the differentiation between active granulomatous inflammation and fibrous lesions.

Patient Preparation for FDG PET for Cardiac Sarcoidosis

Critical factor to FDG PET cardiac sarcoidosis imaging has been to increase the uptake of ^{18}F-FDG by inflammatory cells in myocardium and suppressing physiological cardiomyocyte uptake. The dietary preparation consist of carbohydrate restricted foods for 24 h prior to the test, with an intake of high-fat and high protein foods for at least two meals 24 h prior followed by overnight fast [34–38]. Other method to suppress glucose uptake by normal myocyte include giving IV unfractionated heparin (10 IU/kg 30 min prior + 5 IU/kg 15 min prior or 50 IU/kg 15 min prior to radiotracer administration), resulting in elevated plasma levels of free fatty acids and increasing cardiac utilization of free fatty acids instead of glucose [39, 40] as lower doses of IV heparin appear to be effective in suppressing physiological uptake of ^{18}F-FDG without significant prolongation of partial thromboplastin time.

The interpretation of image pattern varies differently but none have been validated, however several studies correlated that the focal or heterogeneous tracer uptake more correlated with and are characteristic feature of patients with cardiac sarcoidosis [41, 42]. The various studies including a meta-analysis reported sensitivity and specificity of FDG PET/CT in detecting cardiac sarcoidosis between 85–89% and 38–100%, respectively [32, 43, 44].

Due to physiological myocardial glucose uptake, diagnosis of cardiac sarcoidosis often faces challenge with FDG PET/CT, so alternative tracer was evaluated for same. ^{68}Ga-DOTANOC PET/CT study has been explored as an effective alternative with reported accuracy of 100% in one study [45]. In another study, Lapa et al. [46] compared the SSTR-based PET/CT with contrast enhanced MRI (CMR) in detecting cardiac sarcoidosis in suspected patients and the result show sensitivity of 47% for SSTR PET/CT.

4.3.2.3 Others Sites

Grozdic-Milojevic et al. [47] studied bone involvement in chronic active sarcoidosis. Twenty-two percent patient show FDG positive bony lesion with uptake pattern being focal, diffuse and both while CT indicated bone abnormalities in only 5% of the patients. Muscular involvement of sarcoidosis has been described on FDG PET as "tiger man sign" by Soussan et al. [48], which refers to thick linear FDG uptake that predominantly involves the lower legs (2014). Granulomatous bone marrow infiltration in the axial skeleton has been sensitively detected by both FDG PET/CT and MR. Various other studies have also reveal sarcoidosis in multiple other sites like spleen, kidney, muscle, etc.

4.4 Treatment Response Monitoring

Patients demonstrating ambiguous response clinically, serologically, radiologically, or on endoscopy benefit with addition of FDG PET CT showing remission in disease activity. It has been well documented by various studies that corticosteroid therapy shows reduction of FDG uptake than baseline scan, thus proving to be an objective tool of response assessment with the degree of SUV change correlating with clinical and functional improvement [6, 49–51]. (Figs. 4.2 and 4.3; Table 4.2).

Negative FDG PET should be considered for deciding on stopping treatment. Infliximab is an expensive treatment and monitoring response by PET will prove beneficial in deciding to stop treatment. It is imperative that management guided by PET will be economical in the long run with reduction of morbidity and mortality.

Table 4.2 Treatment response evaluation with FDG PET/ CT

Author (year)	Number of patients	PET tracer	Organ	Treatment and conclusion
Keijsers (2008)	12	FDG	Lungs	6# infliximab; SUV decrease, vital capacity, clinical follow up. Decrease in SUVmax of the lung parenchyma correlated with an improvement of vital capacity VC& clinical improvement
Osborne (2014)	23	Rb, FDG	Heart	Corticosteroids, ACE/ARB. Reduction in the intensity and extent of myocardial inflammation on FDG PET was associated with improvement in EF

One specific aspect of benefit of early response evaluation was highlighted by Aide et al. These investigators suggested that early FDG PET/CT can be undertaken within 10 weeks following corticosteroid treatment in individuals with suspected sarcoidosis and/or malignancy the results of early response were able to differentiate between sarcoidosis and neoplastic lesions which would resolve post-treatment [50]. This is beneficial in those cancer patients where active management is not being immediately considered, and FDG PET/CT images show discordant and surplus lesions.

4.5   Role in Chronic Sarcoidosis

A prospective study by Sobic-Saranovic et al. in 90 patients with chronic sarcoidosis demonstrated FDG PET/CT played a significant influencing factor in change in therapy management. FDG PET detected active inflammation in 82% of the patients, 51% of which have normal ACE level and resulted in treatment alteration in 81% of patients with chronic active sarcoidosis [52].

4.6   Prediction and Detection of Relapse

Two studies have evaluated the role of FDG PET/CT in detecting the chances of relapse in patient with sarcoidosis and the study concluded that the patients who were non-responders on FDG PET/CT after completion of therapy and those with high pre-therapy SUV value were independent factor favouring high possibility of relapse [53, 54].

4.7   Disease Prognostication

Diffuse uptake in lungs was earlier thought to indicate poor pulmonary function. However, no prospective studies have demonstrated conclusively any direct relationship of FDG uptake and pulmonary function post-treatment. Pulmonary and cardiac function improvement is a desirable outcome of therapy. However, at present, serial tests are often performed to document treatment response and organ function recovery.

4.8   Current Limitations and Future Directions

Due to the non-specificity of FDG in malignancy and infection or inflammation with non-specific uptake pattern, it is difficult to diagnose sarcoidosis solely on the basis of FDG PET study. Cardiac PET-MR and the in vivo imaging by various tracers could help in understanding the pathophysiology and furthering individualisation of treatment. If specific characteristics on PET/CT or PET-MR could predict the function recovery post-treatment a priori, then treatment could be accordingly tailored to improve outcome.

Key Points

- Sarcoidosis is an intriguing multi-systemic disease of unknown aetiology.

- PET/CT has been studied extensively as an additional imaging tool in the diagnostic armamentarium in the domain of sarcoidosis.

- FDG PET/CT are useful for detecting thoracic disease, extra-thoracic and occult sites and useful in assessing inflammatory activity and extent.

- The sensitivity of ^{18}F-FDG PET has been reported 100% for pulmonary sites and 90% for extra-pulmonary sites.

- FDG PET/CT is not the modality of choice for diagnosis or screening purposes, however, can be utilized after the routine investigations fail to provide adequate diagnosis.

- FDG PET/CT can be useful as a baseline test to document active sites of sarcoidosis in patients with strong clinical suspicion but negative serological markers.

- FDG PET/CT imaging may serve as a non-invasive tool to narrow down differentials and also to increase the yield of biopsy. FDG uptake can mimic the lymph node involvement by malignancy; hence, histological confirmation is mandatory.

- FDG PET/CT may show diffuse or multi-focal uptake pattern, but the severity of pulmonary involvement as assessed by HRCT features and lung function parameters correlated with the PET activity in sarcoidosis.

- Most commonly involved group of lymph nodes in sarcoidosis is mediastinal and hilar lymph nodes but enlarged lymph nodes are not exclusive of sarcoidosis as several conditions like tuberculosis or malignancy can present with lymphadenopathy.

- Combined use of FDG PET/CT and cardiac MR would provide the best results in cardiac sarcoidosis that could allow the differentiation between active granulomatous inflammation and fibrous lesions.

- The interpretation of image pattern varies differently, sensitivity and specificity of FDG PET/CT in detecting cardiac sarcoidosis is between 85–89% and 38–100%, respectively.

- Due to physiological myocardial glucose uptake, diagnosis of cardiac sarcoidosis often faces challenge with FDG PET/CT, so alternative tracer was evaluated for same. ^{68}Ga-DOTANOC PET/CT study has been explored as an effective alternative with reported accuracy of 100% in one study.

- Corticosteroid therapy shows reduction of FDG uptake than baseline scan, thus proving to be an objective tool of response assessment with the degree of SUV change correlating with clinical and functional.

References

1. Statement on sarcoidosis. Joint Statement of the American Thoracic Society (ATS), the European Respiratory Society (ERS) and the World Association of Sarcoidosis and Other Granulomatous Disorders (WASOG) adopted by the ATS Board of Directors and by the ERS Executive Committee, February 1999. Am J Respir Crit Care Med. 1999;160:736–55.
2. Braun JJ, Kessler R, Constantinesco A, Imperiale A. 18F-FDG PET/CT in sarcoidosis management: review and report of 20 cases. Eur J Nucl Med Mol Imaging. 2008;35:1537–43.
3. Keijsers RG, Grutters JC, Thomeer M, et al. Imaging the inflammatory activity of sarcoidosis: sensitivity and inter observer agreement of (67)Ga imaging and (18)F-FDG PET. Q J Nucl Med Mol Imaging. 2011;55:66–71.
4. Nishiyama Y, Yamamoto Y, Fukunaga K, et al. Comparative evaluation of 18F-FDG PET and 67Ga scintigraphy in patients with sarcoidosis. J Nucl Med. 2006;47:1571–6.
5. Lewis PJ, Salama A. Uptake of fluorine-18-fluorodeoxyglucose in sarcoidosis. J Nucl Med. 1994;35:1647–9.
6. Teirstein AS, Machac J, Almeida O, et al. Results of 188 whole-body fluorodeoxyglucose positron emission tomography scans in 137 patients with sarcoidosis. Chest. 2007;132:1949–53.
7. Sobic-Saranovic D, Grozdic I, Videnovic-Ivanov J, et al. The utility of 18F-FDGPET/CT for diagnosis and adjustment of therapy in patients with active chronic sarcoidosis. J Nucl Med. 2012;53:1543–9.
8. Keijsers RG, Verzijlbergen FJ, Oyen WJ, van den Bosch JM, Ruven HJ, van Velzen-Blad H, Grutters JC. 18F-FDG PET, genotype-corrected ACE and sIL-2R in newly diagnosed sarcoidosis. Eur J Nucl Med Mol Imaging. 2009;36(7):1131–7.
9. Dalma VA, van hagen PM, van Koetsveld PM, et al. Expression of somatostatin, cortistatin, and somatostatin receptors in human monocytes, macrophages, and dendritic cells. Am J Physiol Endocrinol Metab. 2003;285:E344–53.
10. ten Bokum AM, Hofland LJ, de Jong G, et al. Immunohistochemical localization of somatostatin receptor in sst2A in sarcoid granuloma. Eur J Clin Investig. 1999;29:630–6.
11. Soydal C, Kucuk O, Ozkan E, Kumbasar O, Kir M. Ga-68 DOTATATE accumulation in sarcoidosis. Int J Nucl Medi Res. 2015;2:1–4.
12. Nobashi T, Nakamoto Y, Kubo T, Ishimori T, Handa T, Tanizawa K, Sano K, Mishima M, Togashi K. The utility of PET/CT with (68)Ga-DOTATOC in sarcoidosis: comparison with (67)Ga-scintigraphy. Ann Nucl Med. 2016;30(8):544–52.
13. Judson MA, Baughman RP, Teirstein AS, et al. Defining organ involvement in sarcoidosis: the ACCESS proposed instrument. Sarcoidosis Vasc Diffuse Lung Dis. 1999;16:75–86.
14. Keir G, Wells AU. Assessing pulmonary disease and response to therapy: which test? Semin Respir Crit Care Med. 2010;31:409–18.
15. Baughman RP, Culver DA, Judson MA. A concise review of pulmonary sarcoidosis. Am J Respir Crit Care Med. 2011;183:573–81.
16. Drent M, De Vries J, Lenters M, et al. Sarcoidosis: assessment of disease severity using HRCT. Eur Radiol. 2003;13:2462–71.
17. Abehsera M, Valeyre D, Grenier P, et al. Sarcoidosis with pulmonary fibrosis: CT patterns and correlation with pulmonary function. AJR Am J Roentgenol. 2000;174:1751–7.
18. Mostard RL, Verschakelen JA, van Kroonenburgh MJ, Nelemans PJ, Wijnen PA, Vöö S, Drent M. Severity of pulmonary involvement and (18)F-FDG PET activity in sarcoidosis. Respir Med. 2013;107(3):439–47.
19. Brudin LH, Valind SO, Rhodes CG, Pantin CF, Sweatman M, Jones T, Hughes JM. Fluorine-18 deoxyglucose uptake in sarcoidosis measured with positron emission tomography. Eur J Nucl Med. 1994;21(4):297–305.
20. Keijsers RG, Verzijlbergen EJ, van den Bosch JM, Zanen P, van de Garde EM, Oyen WJ, Grutters JC. 18F-FDG PET as a predictor of pulmonary function in sarcoidosis. Sarcoidosis Vasc Diffuse Lung Dis. 2011;28(2):123–9.

21. Basu S, Yadav M, Joshi JM, Desai D, Moghe S. Active pre-treatment purepulmonary parenchymal sarcoidosis with raised serum angiotensin converting enzyme level: characteristics on PET with glucose metabolism and cell proliferation tracers and HRCT. Eur J Nucl Med Mol Imaging. 2011;38(8):1584–5.
22. Rayamajhi SJ, Mittal BR, Maturu VN, Agarwal R, Bal A, Dey P, Shukla J, Gupta D. (18) F-FDG and (18)F-FLT PET/CT imaging in the characterization of mediastinal lymph nodes. Ann Nucl Med. 2016;30(3):207–16.
23. Koo HJ, Kim MY, Shin SY, Shin S, Kim SS, Lee SW, Choi CM. Evaluation of mediastinal lymph nodes in sarcoidosis, sarcoid reaction, and malignant lymph nodes using CT and FDG-PET/CT. Medicine (Baltimore). 2015;94(27):e1095.
24. Iwai K, Tachibana Y, Takemura T, Matsui Y, Kitaichi M, Kawabata Y. Pathological studies on sarcoidosis autopsy. I. Epidemiological features of 320 cases in Japan. Acta Pathol Jpn. 1993;43(7–8):372–6.
25. Perry A, Vuitch F. Causes of death in patients with sarcoidosis. A morphologic study of 38 autopsies with clinicopathologic correlations. Arch Pathol Lab Med. 1995;119(2):167–72.
26. Greulich S, Deluigi CC, Gloekler S, Wahl A, Zürn C, Kramer U, et al. CMR imaging predicts death and other adverse events in suspected cardiac sarcoidosis. JACC Cardiovasc Imaging. 2013;6:501–11.
27. Koiwa H, Tsujino I, Ohira H, Yoshinaga K, Otsuka N, Nishimura M. Images in cardiovascular medicine: imaging of cardiac sarcoid lesions using fasting cardiac 18F- fluorodeoxyglucose-positron emission tomography: an autopsy case. Circulation. 2010;122:535–6.
28. Hiraga H, Hiroe M, Iwai K, et al. Guideline for diagnosis of cardiac sarcoidosis: study report on diffuse pulmonary diseases. Tokyo: The Japanese Ministry of Health and Welfare; 1993. p. 23–4. in Japanese.
29. Diagnostic standard and guidelines for sarcoidosis. Jpn J Sarcoidosis Granulomatous Disord. 2007;27:89–102.
30. Schatka I, Bengel FM. Advanced imaging of cardiac sarcoidosis. J Nucl Med. 2014;55:99–106.
31. Skali H, Schulman AR, Dorbala S. 18F-FDG PET/CT for the assessment of myocardial sarcoidosis. Curr Cardiol Rep. 2013;15:352.
32. Youssef G, Leung E, Mylonas I, Nery P, Williams K, Wisenberg G, et al. The use of 18F-FDG PET in the diagnosis of cardiac sarcoidosis: a systematic review and metaanalysis including the Ontario experience. J Nucl Med. 2012;53:241–8.
33. Birnie D. HRS expert consensus statement on the diagnosis and management of arrhythmias associated with cardiac sarcoidosis. Heart Rhythm. 2014;11:1305–23.
34. Langah R, Spicer K, Gebregziabher M, Gordon L. Effectiveness of prolonged fasting 18F-FDG PET-CT in the detection of cardiac sarcoidosis. J Nucl Cardiol. 2009;16:801–10.
35. Harisankar CN, Mittal BR, Agrawal KL, Abrar ML, Bhattacharya A. Utility of high fat and low carbohydrate diet in suppressing myocardial FDG uptake. J Nucl Cardiol. 2011;18:926–36.
36. Williams G, Kolodny GM. Suppression of myocardial 18F-FDG uptake by preparing patients with a high-fat, low-carbohydrate diet. AJR Am J Roentgenol. 2008;190:W151–6.
37. Lum DP, Wandell S, Ko J, Coel MN. Reduction of myocardial 2-deoxy-2-[18F] fluoro-d-glucose uptake artifacts in positron emission tomography using dietary carbohydrate restriction. Mol Imaging Biol. 2002;4:232–7.
38. Persson E. Lipoprotein lipase, hepatic lipase and plasma lipolytic activity. Effects of heparin and a low molecular weight heparin fragment (Fragmin). Acta Med Scand. 1988;724:1–56.
39. Manabe O, Yoshinaga K, Ohira H, Masuda A, Sato T, Tsujino I, et al. The effects of 18-h fasting with low-carbohydrate diet preparation on suppressed physiological myocardial 18F-fluorodeoxyglucose (FDG) uptake and possible minimal effects of unfractionated heparin use in patients with suspected cardiac involvement sarcoidosis. J Nucl Cardiol. 2015;23:244–52.
40. Asmal AC, Leary WP, Thandroyen F, Botha J, Wattrus S. A doseresponse study of the anticoagulant and lipolytic activities of heparin in normal subjects. Br J Clin Pharmacol. 1979;7:531–3.

41. Ishimaru S, Tsujino I, Takei T, Tsukamoto E, Sakaue S, Kamigaki M, Ito N, Ohira H, Ikedo D, Tamaki N, Nishimura M. Focal uptake on 18F-fluoro-2-deoxyglucose positron emission tomography images indicates cardiac involvement of sarcoidosis. Eur Heart J. 2005;26(15):1538–43.

42. Tahara N, Tahara A, Nitta Y, Kodama N, Mizoguchi M, Kaida H, Baba K, Ishibashi M, Hayabuchi N, Narula J, Imaizumi T. Heterogeneous myocardial FDG uptake and the disease activity in cardiac sarcoidosis. JACC Cardiovasc Imaging. 2010;3(12):1219–28.

43. Norikane T, Yamamoto Y, Maeda Y, Noma T, Dobashi H, Nishiyama Y. Comparative evaluation of (18)F-FLT and (18)F-FDG for detecting cardiac and extra-cardiac thoracic involvement in patients with newly diagnosed sarcoidosis. EJNMMI Res. 2017;7(1):69.

44. Ohira H, Tsujino I, Ishimaru S, Oyama N, Takei T, Tsukamoto E, Miura M, Sakaue S, Tamaki N, Nishimura M. Myocardial imaging with 18F-fluoro-2-deoxyglucose positron emission tomography and magnetic resonance imaging in sarcoidosis. Eur J Nucl Med Mol Imaging. 2008;35(5):933–41.

45. Gormsen LC, Haraldsen A, Kramer S, Dias AH, Kim WY, Borghammer P. A dual tracer (68) Ga-DOTANOC PET/CT and (18)F-FDG PET/CT pilot study for detection of cardiac sarcoidosis. EJNMMI Res. 2016;6(1):52.

46. Lapa C, Reiter T, Kircher M, Schirbel A, Werner RA, Pelzer T, Pizarro C, Skowasch D, Thomas L, Schlesinger-Irsch U, Thomas D, Bundschuh RA, Bauer WR, Gärtner FC. Somatostatin receptor based PET/CT in patients with the suspicion of cardiac sarcoidosis: an initial comparison to cardiac MRI. Oncotarget. 2016;7(47):77807–14.

47. Grozdic Milojevic I, Sobic-Saranovic D, Videnovic-Ivanov J, Saranovic D, Odalovic S, Artiko V. FDG PET/CT in bone sarcoidosis. Sarcoidosis Vasc Diffuse Lung Dis. 2016;33(1):66–74.

48. Soussan M, Augier A, Brillet PY, Weinmann P, Valeyre D. Functional imaging in extrapulmonary sarcoidosis: FDG-PET/CT and MR features. Clin Nucl Med. 2014;39(2):e146–59.

49. Zhuang H, Alavi A. 18-fluorodeoxyglucose positron emission tomographic imaging in the detection and monitoring of infection and inflammation. Semin Nucl Med. 2002;32(1):47–59.

50. Aide N, Allouache D, Ollivier Y, de Raucourt S, Switsers O, Bardet S. Early 2′-deoxy-2′-[18F] fluoro-D-glucose PET metabolic response after corticosteroid therapy to differentiate cancer from sarcoidosis and sarcoid-like lesions. Mol Imaging Biol. 2009;11(4):224–8.

51. Keijsers RG, Verzijlbergen JF, van Diepen DM, van den Bosch JM, Grutters JC. 18F-FDG PET in sarcoidosis: an observational study in 12 patients treated with infliximab. Sarcoidosis Vasc Diffuse Lung Dis. 2008;25(2):143–9.

52. Sobic-Saranovic D, Grozdic I, Videnovic-Ivanov J, Vucinic-Mihailovic V, Artiko V, Saranovic D, Djuric-Stefanovic A, Masulovic D, Odalovic S, Ilic-Dudvarski A, Popevic S, Pavlovic S, Obradovic V. The utility of 18F-FDG PET/CT for diagnosis and adjustment of therapy in patients with active chronic sarcoidosis. J Nucl Med. 2012;53(10):1543–9.

53. Vorselaars AD, Verwoerd A, van Moorsel CH, Keijsers RG, Rijkers GT, Grutters JC. Prediction of relapse after discontinuation of infliximab therapy in severe sarcoidosis. Eur Respir J. 2014;43(2):602–9.

54. Maturu VN, Rayamajhi SJ, Agarwal R, Aggarwal AN, Gupta D, Mittal BR. Role of serial F-18 FDG PET/CT scans in assessing treatment response and predicting relapses in patients with symptomatic sarcoidosis. Sarcoidosis Vasc Diffuse Lung Dis. 2016;33(4):372–80.

55. Tirpude S, Basu S, Joshi JM. FDG-PET scan in management of pulmonary sarcoidosis. J Assoc Physicians India. 2013;61(4):276.

56. Basu S, Asopa RV, Baghel NS. Early documentation of therapeutic response at 6 weeks following corticosteroid therapy in extensive sarcoidosis: promise of FDG-PET. Clin Nucl Med. 2009;34(10):689–90.

FDG PET/CT in Assessment of Prosthetic Joint Infection

5

Pradeep Thapa, Ashwini Kalshetty, and Sandip Basu

Contents

5.1   Introduction

In recent years, there is increasing number of individuals undergoing joint replacement surgery owing to increased survival and modern lifestyle. The commonly performed joint replacement surgeries involve the weight bearing hip and knee joints and they significantly reduce the pain and stiffness along with improvement in mobility and quality of life. However, prosthetic joint infection (PJI) is one of the most severe complications; the infection rate after arthroplasty is ~1–2% in lower limbs and almost triples after revision surgery. The cause of implant failure could be either peri-prosthetic infection or aseptic loosening (more common) and hence,

P. Thapa
Radiation Medicine Centre, Bhabha Atomic Research Centre, Tata Memorial Centre Annexe, Mumbai, India

A. Kalshetty · S. Basu (✉)
Radiation Medicine Centre, Bhabha Atomic Research Centre, Tata Memorial Centre Annexe, Mumbai, India

Homi Bhabha National Institute, Mumbai, India

© Springer International Publishing AG, part of Springer Nature 2018
T. Wagner, S. Basu (eds.), *PET/CT in Infection and Inflammation*,
Clinicians' Guides to Radionuclide Hybrid Imaging,
https://doi.org/10.1007/978-3-319-90412-2_5

43

Table 5.1 Definition for periprosthetic joint infection by MSIS (Adapted from Parvizi et al. [6])

Major	Two positive cultures with phenotypically same organism
	A sinus tract communicating with the joint
Minor	High CRP and ESR
	High synovial fluid WBCs or leucocyte esterase test strip and change
	High synovial fluid PMNs
	Periprothetic tissue with positive HPE
	A single positive culture

CRP C reactive protein, *ESR* erythrocyte sedimentation rate, *HPE* histopathological examination

correct diagnosis is critical for timely management and good outcome. The mortality rate due to prosthetic joint infections is 2.5% and these infections are also associated with morbidity, disability, and cost implications. The management of PJI almost always necessitates the need for surgical intervention and prolonged courses of intravenous or oral antimicrobial therapy [1–4] where as aseptic loosening requires less aggressive management compared to the PJI.

There have been a number of parameters taken into consideration while diagnosing PJI. In one of the early prospective case control study by Berbari et al., risk factors for the development of prosthetic joint infection were studied [5]. The proposed criteria for prediction of PJIs: (a) postoperative surgical site infection, (b) national nosocomial infection surveillance score >2.0, (c) concurrent malignancy, and (d) prior THA.

The Workgroup of the Musculoskeletal Infection Society (MSIS) proposed the new definition for peri-prosthetic joint infection as follows (Table 5.1) [6].

5.2   FDG PET/CT in PJI

The routine clinical or laboratory tests have low sensitivity, specificity, and accuracy for the diagnosis of prosthetic joint infection. Hence, a combination of laboratory investigations, histopathology, microbiology, and imaging studies is frequently required [7]. The blood leukocyte count and differential is not sufficiently discriminative or cannot convincingly predict either the presence or absence of infection [1]. Synovial fluid leukocyte count of $>1.7 \times 10^9/L$ and differential of >65% neutrophils was reported to have a sensitivity for diagnosing PJI of 94% and 97%, and specificity of 88% and 98%, respectively [8]. Histopathological examination has sensitivity of >80% and a specificity >90% [7]. However, the degree of infiltration with inflammatory cells may vary considerably between specimens from the same patient, even within individual tissue sections. Therefore, areas with the most florid inflammatory changes should be assessed and at least ten high-power fields should be examined to obtain an average count [9]. The methods of culture and sensitivity also demonstrate false-negative and false-positive results in a considerable number of cases. More recently, several new tools have been investigated such as (a) use of proteomics and analyzing synovial fluid biomarkers (α-defensin, IL-6, and CRP), (b) visualizing biofilms with fluorescent in situ hybridization and detection of bacteria via DNA microarray (for bettering culture-sensitivity results), and (c) use of amplification-based molecular techniques in cases of culture-negative PJI [10].

As each modality continues to demonstrate limitations, there has been endeavours to explore the feasibility of the newer noninvasive imaging modality like ^{18}F-fluoro-2-deoxy-D-glucose positron emission tomography (FDG PET and PET/CT) in management of PJIs in view of its great promise shown in the evaluation of infection and inflammation [11, 12]. Not only being technically less demanding, it scores many points over routine radiolabelled leucocyte-marrow (WBC/BM) imaging like easy availability, short duration of study period and safe with lower radiation exposure. PET also provides superior spatial resolution compared to the WBC/BM imaging, and hence may provide an advantage in managing these patients [12, 13].

Several previous studies have laid down the criteria for differentiating infected prosthesis from non-infected one (Table 5.2).

The various criteria for peri-prosthetic infection on FDG PET or PET/CT used in different studies were based on:

1. Visual assessment
2. Semi-quantitative analyses: dividing the bone–prosthesis interface into segments and giving each segment a score.
3. Quantitative parameters like SUVmax

Among these, the visual interpretation has stood the test of time and by far has come close to the accurate diagnosis in hip and knee arthroplasty-related infection. Single semi-quantitative parameter-like SUVmax has not shown any reproducible results for PJIs.

Table 5.2 Criteria for PJI on FDG PET/CT

Author	Criteria for infection on FDG PET	Final diagnosis
Chryssikos et al. [15]	FDG uptake at bone-prosthesis interface of the femoral component	(1) open wound or sinus in communication with the joint;(2) a systemic infection with pain in the hip and purulent fluid within the joint; or (3) a positive result on at least three tests (ESR, CRP, joint aspiration, intraoperative frozen section, and intraoperative culture)
Basu et al. [16]	Positivity criteria for infection in THAs: Increased FDG uptake was noted at the prosthesis-bone interface in the middle portion of the shaft of the hip prosthesis. Negative:FDG uptake was limited to the soft tissues, or adjacent only to the neck of the prosthesis. Positive for infection in TKRs: Positive: Only uptake at the bone/prosthesis interface Negative: No or minimal uptake	Microbiological examinations of the surgical specimens in 125 prostheses, joint aspirations, clinical follow-up of 6 months or more in 86 prostheses

(continued)

Table 5.2 (continued)

Author	Criteria for infection on FDG PET	Final diagnosis
Mumme T et al. [17]	Five categories 1. No uptake in interface bone-prosthesis 2. Uptake surrounding femoral neck 3. Uptake localised in the area surrounding the femoral neck and in a part of the bone–acetabular cup and/or I and VII Gruen's zones 4. Uptake in the area surrounding the femoral neck and in the totality of the bone–femoral cup interface, without compromising periprosthetic soft tissue 5. Uptake localised in the neck area and in most of the bone–stem interface without compromising periprosthetic soft tissue 6. IVa plus IVb 7. Uptake in bone–prosthesis interface and in periprosthetic soft tissue	Operative findings, microbiological and histological examinations in symptomatic group Asymptomatic arthroplasties ($n = 20$) were integrated into a clinical follow-up (≥ 9 months)
Delank KS et al. [18]	Increased FDG uptake in the periprosthetic soft tissue	Intra-operative findings, HPE, microbiology
Vanquickenborne B et al. [19]	FDG uptake ≥grade 2 than control group (?)	Microbiology, clinical f/u ≤6 months
Gravius et al. [20]	Interface between bone and surrounding soft tissue/ bone was divided into 3 segments each for both femur & tibia and in addition for 4 segments reflecting the surrounding periprosthetic soft tissue. FDG uptake in each of the segments was scored (0–3)	Operative findings, microbiological culture and histological examination
Chacko et al. [21]	Increased FDG uptake at the BPI (uptake limited to the soft tissues adjacent to the neck or the tip of the femoral component was not considered a sign of infection)	Microbiology, histopathology, surgical findings and clinical follow-up

The criteria include characteristic pattern of uptake and location for infection, like uptake in mid-shaft of the implant at the bone–prosthesis interface (Fig. 5.1). If increased FDG uptake was present in the bone–prosthesis interface for either hip or knee arthroplasty compared with adjacent soft tissue, a diagnosis of infected prosthesis was suggested (Figs. 5.2 and 5.3) and if no such increased tracer uptake was seen, infection was considered unlikely. As for hip prosthesis,

Fig. 5.1 In this patient with bilateral hip prostheses, the maximum intensity projection image shows FDG uptake patterns in non-infected hip prosthesis and infected hip prosthesis. In the right non-infected hip prosthesis, some uptake of FDG is noted around the neck (arrow heads), while the bone-prosthesis interface appears without significant FDG uptake. In contrast, the left infected hip prosthesis reveals significant tracer concentration at the bone-prosthesis interface (arrows). In this particular patient, there is also significant activity in the tip of the prosthesis (dashed arrow) (Reproduced with permission from Basu et al. [16])

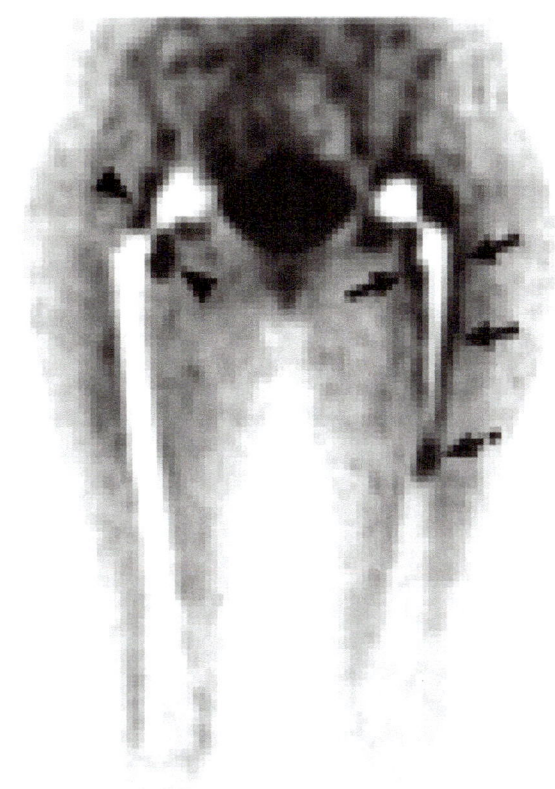

FDG uptake around femoral head and neck can be seen for months or years after the THA. Thus, if the increased tracer uptake is observed around the femoral head or neck portion of the prosthesis but did not extend to the femoral shaft, loosening was considered a likely diagnosis [14, 15] and does not favor a diagnosis of infection.

The literature review searched resulted in various studies evaluating the effectiveness of FDG PET/CT in diagnosing PJI (Table 5.3) and they have included many criteria for infection like FDG uptake at bone–prosthesis interface, dividing uptake into categories ranging from no uptake to uptake in bone–prosthesis interface and in peri-prosthetic soft tissue. The pooled sensitivity, specificity, positive predictive value, negative predictive value from these studies were 82–100%, 79–97%, 69–95%, 90–98%, and 82–91%, respectively [14–21].

A recently published systematic review on the subject demonstrated a pooled sensitivity of 87% and a pooled specificity of 87% in diagnosing PJIs by FDG PET/CT [22].

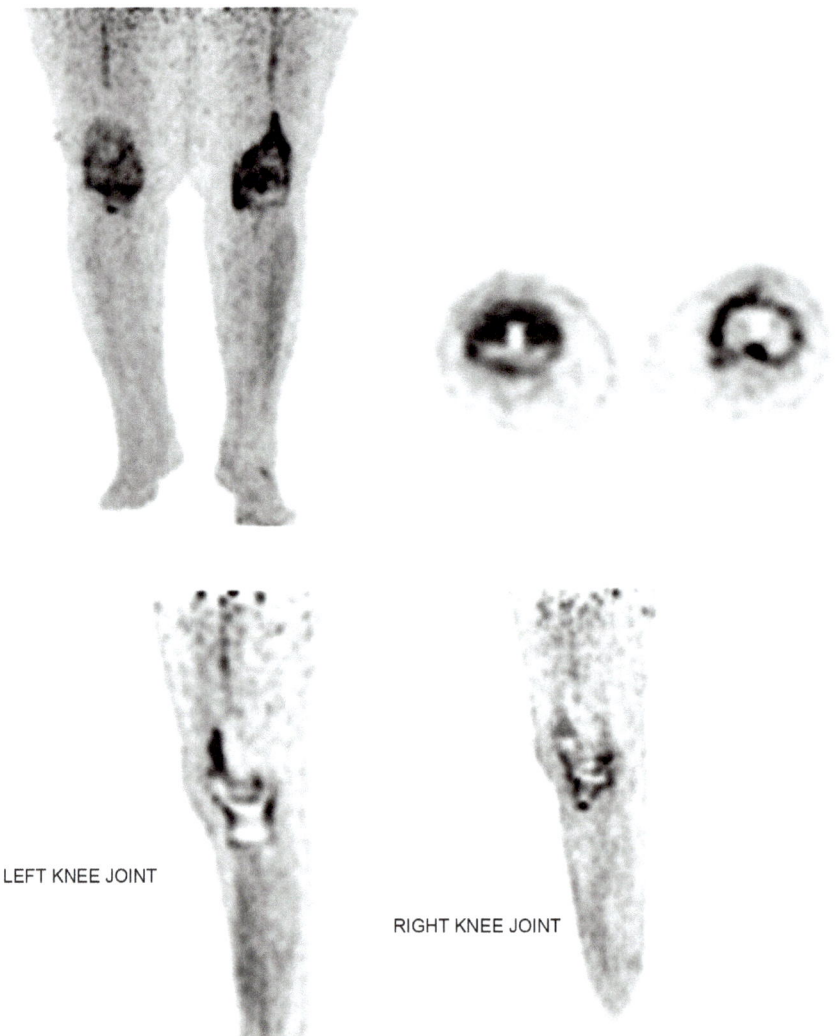

LEFT KNEE JOINT

RIGHT KNEE JOINT

Fig. 5.2 Patient infected bilateral total knee replacement (right knee- 2004, left knee-revision TKR on 2009), with complaints of pain in both knee joints in 2014, more on right knee joint. Both sides are abnormal and suspicious for infection. Tomographic images showed the exact locations of these sites at the bone-prosthesis interface. Uptake in the prosthesis bone interface is a suspect for infection

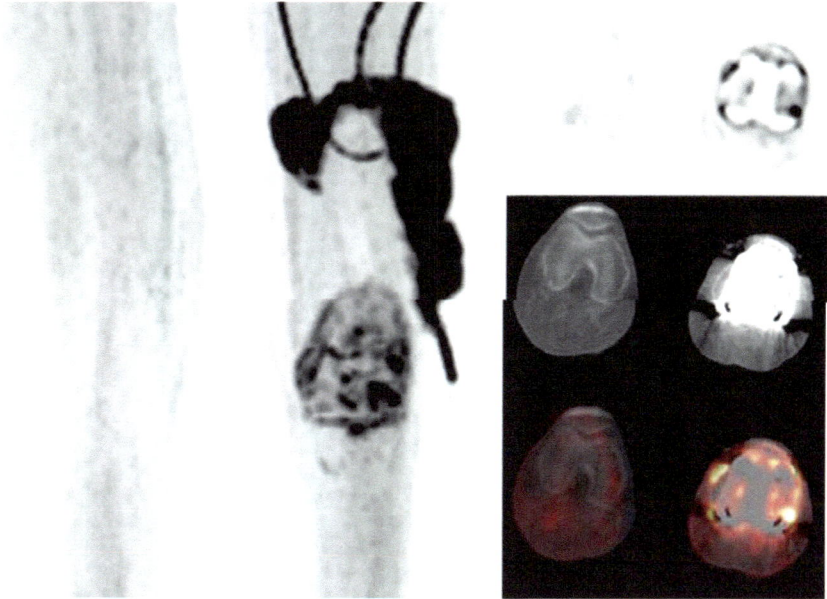

Fig. 5.3   Infected knee prosthesis. Coronal PET *(left column) and* axial PET, CT, and fused PET/CT *(right column) show focally* increased FDG uptake at the prosthesis-bone interfaces of the knee prosthesis as well as more diffuse distribution consistent with synovitis. Note the severe metal induced artefacts on CT (Reproduced with permission from Basu et al. [28])

5.3   Drawbacks of FDG PET

The lower specificity of FDG PET study is due to the nonspecific FDG uptake around prosthesis. Zhuang et al. reported that increased FDG uptake around the femoral head and neck may persist for years following hip arthroplasty and can occur in both symptomatic and asymptomatic patients; likely due to foreign body reaction [23]. Increased FDG uptake around the distal tip of the hip prosthesis is also nonspecific.

Another factor leading to low specificity is due to high FDG concentration around prosthesis due to metallic artifacts in attenuated corrected images [24]. This artifact can be minimized by viewing the non-attenuated corrected images, which should always be compared to remove the ambiguity.

Table 5.3 Performance of FDG PET/CT in diagnosing PJI

Author	Study type	Total patients	Total joints	THA/TKR	Diagnostic criteria	Sn/Sp/PPV/NPV (%)
Chryssikos et al. [15]	Prospective	113	127	+/−	Increased FDG activity at the bone-prosthesis interface of the femoral component.	85/93/80/95
Basu et al. [16]	Prospective	221	221	+/+	Abnormal FDG uptake along the bone prosthesis interface in the middle portion of the shaft of the hip prosthesis and for the patients with knee arthroplasty, only uptake at the bone/prosthesis interface was considered as being consistent with infection.	81.8/93.1/79.4/94 for hip prosthesis 94.7/88.2/69.2/98.4 for knee prosthesis
Mumme et al. [17]	Prospective	50	70	+/−	Five categories 1. No uptake in interface bone-prosthesis 2. Uptake surrounding femoral neck 3. Uptake localised in the area surrounding the femoral neck and in a part of the bone–acetabular cup and/or I and VII Gruen's zones 4. Uptake in the area surrounding the femoral neck and in the totality of the bone–femoral cup interface, without compromising periprosthetic soft tissue 5. Uptake localised in the neck area and in most of the bone–stem interface without compromising periprosthetic soft tissue 6. IVa plus IVb 7. Uptake in bone–prosthesis interface and in periprosthetic soft tissue	91/92/−/−
Vanquickenborne B et al. [19]	Prospective	17	17	+/−	FDG uptake ≥grade 2 than control group (?)	88/78/−/−
Chacko et al. [21]	Prospective	32	41	+/−	Increased FDG uptake at the BPI (uptake limited to the soft tissues adjacent to the neck or the tip of the femoral component was not considered a sign of infection)	91.7/96.6/95.1/−

Nonspecific uptake in healing tissues could last up to 6 months post-surgery. Because of nonspecific FDG uptake in postoperative site in healing phase, the clinical role of early PET CT is questionable. Most studies have PET CT done after 6 months of surgery. Prospective studies are needed to observe patterns of uptake in asymptomatic and in early period following surgery. Zhuang et al. noted FDG uptake minimizes by 3 months of surgery. Nonetheless, many studies in symptomatic cases after 6 months show high performance of FDG PET CT in diagnosing PJIs.

5.4 Beyond FDG: FDG-Labelled Leukocyte Imaging

FDG-labelled WBCs could be considered as alternative to noninvasive diagnosis of PJI as study have demonstrated that 87% of ^{18}F-FDG incubated with a WBC pellet is found in granulocytes [25]. Two studies with FDG-labelled leukocyte in PJI have shown pooled sensitivity, specificity, positive predictive, and negative predictive value of 86–93%, 86–97%, 86–93%, and 97–100% [25, 26]. The concerns of FDG-labelled WBCs include labelling yield, labelled leukocyte load, blood formula, and propensity for homing in the reticuloendothelial system [27].

Potential indications of PET in patients of PJIs include:

(a) Noninvasive diagnosis of PJI with localization
(b) Guide biopsy for increasing yield
(c) Response assessment (could be monitored FDG-positive PJIs)
(d) Occult site of infection
(e) Risk stratification through assessment of involvement of joint space, stability of joint/prosthesis, the integrity of surrounding soft tissue.

Conclusion

The indications and potential use of PET have not been explored fully. Most studies have compared the accuracy of FDG PET/CT with other biological and radiological markers. However, FDG PET CT can also guide tissue biopsy or aspiration to increase the yield and towards accurate diagnosis. Extra information can be actively sought for instead of just classifying into infection present or not and include the presence of periosteal reaction, peri-prosthetic osteolysis, peri-prosthetic calcification, sinus tract description, localization of infection, extent of infection, involvement of joint space, stability of joint/prosthesis, the integrity of surrounding soft tissue, etc. which can be of additional value in guiding the orthopedic surgeon in the management of these patients. If PJI is due to hematogenous spread of infection then, FDG PET/CT may additionally help in localization of distant source of infection. The heterogeneity of criteria, lack of specificity in diagnosis, and relatively lower yield of PET studies suggest that they should be examined further by larger prospective trials.

Key Points

- FDG PET/CT is useful in management of PJIs (technically less demanding, easy availability, short duration of study period and safe with lower radiation exposure).

- PET provides superior spatial resolution compared to the WBC/BM imaging, and hence may provide an advantage in managing these patients.

- There are various criteria for evaluation of peri-prosthetic infection on FDG PET or PET/CT. Visual interpretation is found to be accurate in diagnoses of hip and knee arthroplasty-related infection.

- Increased FDG uptake at the bone–prosthesis interface for either hip or knee arthroplasty compared with adjacent soft tissue, a diagnosis of infected prosthesis was suggested.

- FDG uptake around femoral head and neck can be seen for months or years after the hip arthroplasty.

- The lower specificity of FDG PET study is due to the nonspecific FDG uptake around prosthesis.

- Increased FDG uptake around the femoral head and neck may persist for years following hip arthroplasty and can occur in both symptomatic and asymptomatic patients; likely due to foreign body reaction.

- Increased FDG uptake around the distal tip of the hip prosthesis is also nonspecific.

- High FDG concentration around prosthesis due to metallic artifacts in attenuated corrected images limits specificity, but viewing non-attenuated corrected images, may remove the ambiguity.

- Nonspecific uptake in healing tissues could last up to 6 months post-surgery. Because of nonspecific FDG uptake in postoperative site in healing phase, the clinical role of early PET/CT is questionable.

References

1. Steckelberg JM, Osmon DR. Prosthetic joint infections. In: Waldvogel FAB, Bisno AL, editors. Infections associated with indwelling medical devices. 3rd ed. Washington, DC: American Society for Microbiology; 2000. p. 173–209.
2. Zimmerli W, Trampuz A, Ochsner PE. Prosthetic-joint infections. N Engl J Med. 2004;351:1645–54.
3. Darouiche RO. Treatment of infections associated with surgical implants. N Engl J Med. 2004;350:1422–9.

4. Sia IG, Berbari EF, Karchmer AW. Prosthetic joint infections. Infect Dis Clin N Am. 2005;19:885–914.
5. Berbari EF, Hanssen AD, Duffy MC, Steckelberg JM, Ilstrup DM, Harmsen WS, Osmon DR. Risk factors for prosthetic joint infection: case-control study. Clin Infect Dis. 1998;27(5):1247–54.
6. Parvizi J, Gehrke T, International Consensus Group on Periprosthetic Joint Infection. Definition of periprosthetic joint infection. J Arthroplast. 2014;29(7):1331.
7. Trampuz A, Steckelberg JM, Osmon DR, Cockerill FR, Hanssen AD, Patel R. Advances in the laboratory diagnosis of prosthetic joint infection. Rev Med Microbiol. 2003;14:1–14.
8. Trampuz A, Hanssen AD, Osmon DR, Mandrekar J, Steckelberg JM, Patel R. Synovial fluid leukocyte count and differential for the diagnosis of prosthetic knee infection. Am J Med. 2004;117:556–62.
9. Athanasou NA, Pandey R, de Steiger R, Crook D, Smith PM. Diagnosis of infection by frozen section during revision arthroplasty. J Bone Joint Surg Br. 1995;77:28–33.
10. Patel R, Alijanipour P, Parvizi J. Advancements in diagnosing periprosthetic joint infections after total hip and knee arthroplasty. Open Orthop J. 2016;10:654–61.
11. Basu S, Chryssikos T, Moghadam-Kia S, et al. Positron emission tomography as a diagnostic tool in infection: present role and future possibilities. Semin Nucl Med. 2009;39:36–51.
12. Basu S, Zhuang H, Torigian DA, et al. Functional imaging of inflammatory diseases using nuclear medicine techniques. Semin Nucl Med. 2009;39:124–45.
13. Kwee TC, Basu S, Torigian DA, et al. FDG-PET imaging for diagnosing prosthetic joint infection: discussing the facts, rectifying the unsupported claims and call for evidence-based and scientific approach. Eur J Nucl Med Mol Imaging. 2013;40:464–6.
14. Zhuang H, Duarte PS, Pourdehnad M, Maes A, Van Acker F, Shnier D, Garino JP, Fitzgerald RH, Alavi A. The promising role of 18F-FDG PET in detecting infected lower limb prosthesis implants. J Nucl Med. 2001;42(1):44–8.
15. Chryssikos T, Parvizi J, Ghanem E, Newberg A, Zhuang H, Alavi A. FDG-PET imaging can diagnose periprosthetic infection of the hip. Clin Orthop Relat Res. 2008;466(6):1338–42.
16. Basu S, Kwee TC, Saboury B, Garino JP, Nelson CL, Zhuang H, Parsons M, Chen W, Kumar R, Salavati A, Werner TJ, Alavi A. FDG PET for diagnosing infection in hip and knee prostheses: prospective study in 221 prostheses and subgroup comparison with combined (111) In-labeled leukocyte/(99m)Tc-sulfur colloid bone marrow imaging in 88 prostheses. Clin Nucl Med. 2014;39(7):609–15.
17. Mumme T, Reinartz P, Alfer J, Müller-Rath R, Buell U, Wirtz DC. Diagnostic values of positron emission tomography versus triple-phase bone scan in hip arthroplasty loosening. Arch Orthop Trauma Surg. 2005;125(5):322–9.
18. Delank KS, Schmidt M, Michael JW, Dietlein M, Schicha H, Eysel P. The implications of 18F-FDG PET for the diagnosis of endoprosthetic loosening and infection in hip and knee arthroplasty: results from a prospective, blinded study. BMC Musculoskelet Disord. 2006;7:20.
19. Vanquickenborne B, Maes A, Nuyts J, Van Acker F, Stuyck J, Mulier M, Verbruggen A, Mortelmans L. The value of (18)FDG-PET for the detection of infected hip prosthesis. Eur J Nucl Med Mol Imaging. 2003;30(5):705–15.
20. Gravius S, Gebhard M, Ackermann D, Büll U, Hermanns-Sachweh B, Mumme T. Analysis of 18F-FDG uptake pattern in PET for diagnosis of aseptic loosening versus prosthesis infection after total knee arthroplasty. A prospective pilot study. Nuklearmedizin. 2010;49(3):115–23.
21. Chacko TK, Zhuang H, Stevenson K, Moussavian B, Alavi A. The importance of the location of fluorodeoxyglucose uptake in periprosthetic infection in painful hip prostheses. Nucl Med Commun. 2002;23(9):851–5.
22. Hao R, Yuan L, Kan Y, Yang J. 18F-FDG PET for diagnosing painful arthroplasty/prosthetic joint infection. Clin Transl Imaging. 2017;5(4):315–22. https://doi.org/10.1007/s40336-017-0237-8.

23. Zhuang H, Chacko TK, Hickeson M, Stevenson K, Feng Q, Ponzo F, et al. Persistent non-specific FDG uptake on PET imaging following hip arthroplasty. Eur J Nucl Med Mol Imaging. 2002;29:1328–33.
24. Goerres GW, Ziegler SI, Burger C, Berthold T, Von Schulthess GK, Buck A. Artifacts at PET and PET/CT caused by metallic hip prosthetic material. Radiology. 2003;226(2):577–84.
25. Osman S, Danpure HJ. The use of 2-[^{18}F]fluoro-2-deoxy-D-glucose as a potential in vitro agent for labelling human granulocytes for clinical studies by positron emission tomography. Int J Rad Appl Instrum B. 1992;19:183–90.
26. Dumarey N, Egrise D, Blocklet D, Stallenberg B, Remmelink M, del Marmol V, Van Simaeys G, Jacobs F, Goldman S. Imaging infection with 18F-FDG-labeled leukocyte PET/CT: initial experience in 21 patients. J Nucl Med. 2006;47(4):625–32.
27. Aksoy SY, Asa S, Ozhan M, Ocak M, Sager MS, Erkan ME, Halac M, Kabasakal L, Sönmezoglu K, Kanmaz B. FDG and FDG-labelled leucocyte PET/CT in the imaging of prosthetic joint infection. Eur J Nucl Med Mol Imaging. 2014;41(3):556–64.
28. Basu S, Kwee TC, Hess S. FDG-PET/CT imaging of infected bones and prosthetic joints. Curr Mol Imaging. 2014;3(3):225–9.

FDG PET/CT in Evaluating Osteomyelitis and Diabetic Foot

6

Alok Pawaskar and Sandip Basu

Contents

6.1   Introduction

Osteomyelitis (OM) is defined as an infection of the bone. It can involve any bone and is commonly caused by staphylococcus aureus. OM can be caused by haematogenous route, contiguous spread and iatrogenic or post- traumatic exposure of bone. OM can either be acute or chronic type. Early diagnosis is necessary in order to avoid its complications like loss of function and bone loss or fracture. Typical workup of clinically suspected OM includes leucocyte count, serological inflammatory

A. Pawaskar
Radiation Medicine Centre, Bhabha Atomic Research Centre, Tata Memorial Centre Annexe, Mumbai, India

HCG Manavata Cancer Centre, Nashik, India

S. Basu (✉)
Radiation Medicine Centre, Bhabha Atomic Research Centre, Tata Memorial Centre Annexe, Mumbai, India

Homi Bhabha National Institute, Mumbai, India

© Springer International Publishing AG, part of Springer Nature 2018
T. Wagner, S. Basu (eds.), *PET/CT in Infection and Inflammation*,
Clinicians' Guides to Radionuclide Hybrid Imaging,
https://doi.org/10.1007/978-3-319-90412-2_6

Table 6.1 Advantages of FDG
PET/CT over conventional
radionuclide studies in infection
and inflammation

High sensitivity
High resolution images
High target to background ratio
Fast technique completed in one session

Reprinted from PET Clin 2014;9(4):497–519. Hess et al.
"FDG PET/CT in infectious and inflammatory diseases", with
permission from Elsevier

markers, X-ray, and blood culture. Histopathological examination concludes the
diagnosis. However, none of the tests mentioned are very specific for OM and biopsies are invasive. Conventional radionuclide imaging tests such as bone scintigraphy,
labelled white blood cell (WBC) scintigraphy, and gallium scanning all have the
drawbacks of relatively low spatial resolution; they are time consuming, technically
demanding, need handling of blood products (WBC labelling) and lack of sensitivity,
specificity, or both. FDG PET/CT has several advantages over conventional radionuclide imaging and morphological imaging alone (Table 6.1).

Patients with diabetes mellitus (DM) are prone for developing osteomyelitis
complicating the diabetic foot. Diabetic foot refers to ulceration, infection, and/or
destruction of deep tissues of foot with associated neurological abnormalities and
peripheral vascular disease. In the management of diabetic foot, it is very important
to distinguish soft tissue infections from osteomyelitis and to know the extent of
involvement. Here, FDG PET/CT scores over conventional modalities for accurate
delineation of diabetic foot infections due to its superior resolution.

6.2   Osteomyelitis in Axial and Appendicular Skeleton: Performance of FDG PET/CT

The literature evidence on diagnosis of osteomyelitis using FDG PET/CT estab-
lishes this modality as one of the most promising imaging modality with sensitivity
and specificity more than 90% in most of the studies [1–3]. Although, it is very
sensitive for detection of infection with high negative predictive value, its specificity may be low in immediate post-operative setting. This is because post-operative
inflammation persists up to 4–6 weeks after the procedure. In a meta-analysis done
by Termaat et al. [4], FDG PET showed the highest accuracy in diagnosing and
excluding chronic osteomyelitis, with a sensitivity of 96% and a specificity of 91%,
compared to 78 and 84% with combined bone and leukocyte scintigraphy and 84%
and 60% with magnetic resonance imaging (MRI).

For spinal infections, leukocyte imaging or combination of leukocyte imaging and
bone marrow scan have limited sensitivity as infection may be walled off. MRI is not
a preferable option in patients with metallic implants. FDG PET/CT in patients with
suspected spinal infection with and without metallic implants have shown sensitivities well above 90%, and specificity and accuracy at about 90% [5, 6].

In head-to-head comparison of FDG PET/CT and MRI by Demirev et al., the
investigators observed that both were accurate for diagnosis of active osteomyelitis.
A SUVmax cut-off of three gave optimal results with sensitivity of 88% and

specificity of 90% for FDG PET/CT, whereas SUVmax ratio (i.e. lesion SUVmax divided by SUVmax in a reference region) gave inferior results [7]. The authors concluded that MRI can be considered the primary imaging modality for uncomplicated unifocal cases of osteomyelitis, whereas in cases of suspected multifocal disease or contraindications for MRI, FDG PET/CT should be preferred. This combined sequential strategy worked well particularly for the equivocal cases.

6.3   Infectious Spondylodiscitis

It comprises of about 2–4% of osteomyelitis cases and is mostly seen in patients with fever of unknown origin or as metastatic complication in bacteraemia [8]. CT scan or MRI imaging may be difficult to interpret because of the inability to differentiate degenerative changes and infection. Preliminary studies reported the diagnostic sensitivities of FDG PET/CT to approach 100% and specificities of 75–100%, both at 100% for discriminating degenerative changes from disc-space infection and thereby far surpassing MRI's sensitivity of only 50% [9, 10]. Thus, addition of FDG PET/CT in equivocal MRI findings may reduce the need for surgical exploration [11]. Meta-analysis done by Prodromou et al. from 12 pooled studies found the sensitivity and specificity of FDG PET/CT to be 97% and 88%, respectively, with excellent ability to rule out the diagnosis with a very low negative likelihood ratio of <0.1. Importantly, implants and other confounding factors did not affect the diagnostic efficacy when combined FDG PET/CT was employed [12].

6.4   FDG PET/CT in Diabetic Foot

Diabetic foot is a unique entity caused by diabetic neuropathy or peripheral vascular disease and frequently a combination of both. There is loss of protective sensation and development of anatomical deformities both making the feet susceptible to repetitive trauma and ulceration. These make soft tissues of feet accessible to infective organisms. Further defence and treatment is weakened because the access of protective phagocytic cells and antibiotics is reduced because of impaired circulation related to peripheral vascular disease. Another important entity in the context of DM is neuro-osteoarthropathy or Charcot arthropathy, where non-infectious soft tissue inflammation is associated with rapidly progressive destruction of joints and bone.

The estimated risk of a diabetic patient developing a foot ulcer in his or her lifetime has been proposed to be as high as 25%, and the annual incidence of foot ulcers has been estimated to be up to 2% [13, 14]. In up to one-third of diabetic foot infections, osteomyelitis can supervene and is frequently the result of direct extension of the adjacent soft tissue infection. These happen in approximately 15% of overall diabetic patients [15].

Early diagnosis of infection in diabetic foot is of paramount importance as it is treatable with appropriate antibiotics and can potentially prevent complications needing amputation in some cases. When it comes to soft tissue infection, MRI with its excellent soft tissue delineation is the modality of choice. In a meta-analysis undertaken by Dinh and colleagues [16], they compared role of exposed bone or probe-to-bone test, plain film radiography (PFR), MRI, bone scan and leukocyte scan in detection of infection in diabetic foot. They concluded the presence of exposed bone or a positive probe-to-bone test result is moderately predictive of osteomyelitis and MR imaging is the most accurate imaging test for diagnosis of osteomyelitis. As discussed earlier FDG PET has already established as very sensitive modality in imaging bone infection. Hence, combination of PET/CT and MRI or PET-MRI has potential to become the best imaging combination for investigating suspected osteomyelitis in diabetic foot (Fig. 6.1).

The studies comparing the role of FDG PET or PET/CT in diabetic foot have shown conflicting results (Table 6.2) though the studies undertaken with highest numbers have shown utility of FDG PET in this patient group. One of the largest studies done by Nawaz and colleagues [17] reported results from 110 prospectively investigated diabetic patients. In this study, head-to-head comparison was made between FDG PET, MR imaging, and PFR of the feet. They obtained promising results with FDG PET, which correctly diagnosed osteomyelitis in 21 of 26 patients and correctly excluded it in 74 of 80, with sensitivity, specificity, PPV, NPV, and accuracy of 81%, 93%, 78%, 94%, and 90%, respectively. MR imaging had sensitivity, specificity, PPV, NPV, and accuracy of 91%, 78%, 56%, 97%, and 81%,

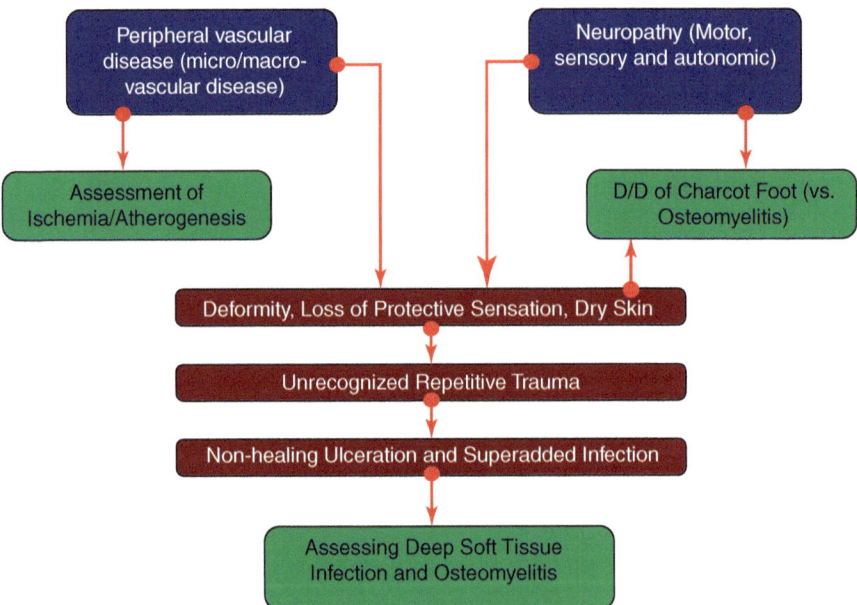

Fig. 6.1 Primary pathogenetic factors (blue); the further complicating factors (brown); in diabetic foot syndrome and diagnostic challenges where PET/CT/PET-MR imaging has a potential role (green). Reprinted from PET Clin, 2012 Apr, 7(2): 151–60, Basu et al. 'FDG PET and PET/CT imaging in complicated diabetic foot'

Table 6.2 Reported studies examining the role of FDG PET/PET/CT in diabetic foot syndrome

Study (first author, year)	No. patients	Charcot arthropathy separately analyzed	PET alone/ PET/CT	Conclusion (useful/ limited accuracy)
Hopfner et al. [14], 2004	16	Yes	PET alone	Useful
Keidar et al. [12], 2005	18	No	PET/CT	Useful
Basu et al. [18], 2007	63	Yes	PET alone	Useful
Schwegler et al. [10], 2008	20	No	PET alone	Limited accuracy
Nawaz et al. [17], 2010	110	No	PET alone	Useful
Familiari et al. [11], 2011	13	No	PET/CT	Limited accuracy

Reprinted from PET Clin, 2012 Apr, 7(2): 151–60, Basu et al. 'FDG PET and PET/CT imaging in complicated diabetic foot'

respectively, while PFR had sensitivity, specificity, PPV, NPV, and accuracy of 63%, 87%, 60%, 88%, and 81%, respectively. The investigators concluded that FDG PET is a highly specific imaging modality for the diagnosis of osteomyelitis in the diabetic foot and, therefore, should be considered to be a useful complementary imaging modality with MR imaging.

Clinically, it is very important to differentiate between osteomyelitis and Charcot arthropathy as management of these two conditions is vastly different. Another large prospective study by Basu and colleagues [18] also showed promising results in diagnosing osteomyelitis and differentiating it from Charcot foot. A low degree of diffuse FDG uptake that was clearly distinguishable from that of normal joints was observed in joints of patients with Charcot osteoarthropathy (Fig. 6.2). The SUVmax in lesions of patients with Charcot osteoarthropathy varied from 0.7 to 2.4, whereas those of the mid foot of the healthy control subjects and the uncomplicated diabetic foot ranged from 0.2 to 0.7 and from 0.2 to 0.8, respectively. The only patient with Charcot osteoarthropathy with superimposed osteomyelitis in this series had an SUVmax of 6.5. The SUVmax of the sites of osteomyelitis as a complication of diabetic foot was 2.9–6.2. The overall sensitivity and accuracy of FDG PET in the diagnosis of Charcot osteoarthropathy were 100.0% and 93.8%, respectively, and those for MR imaging were 76.9% and 75.0%, respectively. The investigators concluded that these results underscored the valuable role of FDG PET in the setting of Charcot neuroarthropathy by reliably differentiating it from osteomyelitis, both in general and when foot ulcer is present.

The ischemic component in development of diabetic foot cannot be ignored. FDG PET, by its ability to assess atherosclerotic inflammation in the large vessels may be able to access this. However, this area in diabetic foot is not yet fully explored and very few studies have explored this area [19, 20]. There is need for further studies in this regard.

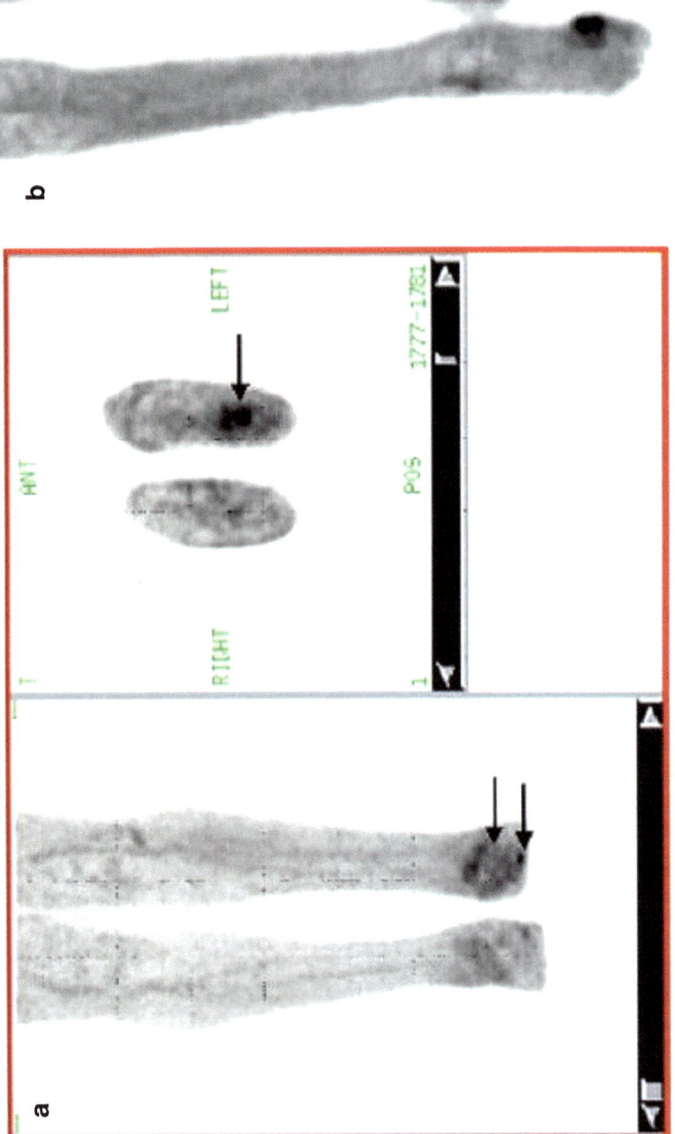

Fig. 6.2 (**a**) FDG PET in a patient with diabetes mellitus demonstrating focal uptake in the ulcer (arrows) in the transaxial images and the relatively low grade diffuse uptake in the neuropathic osteoarthropathy (arrows) are clearly distinguishable from the uptake observed on the unaffected contra lateral limb by visual inspection. (**b**) High grade FDG uptake clearly distinctive from that of Charcot's neuroarthropathy. Reprinted from Basu S, Chryssikos T, Houseni M, et al. Potential role of FDG PET in the setting of diabetic neuroosteoarthropathy: can it differentiate uncomplicated Charcot's neuropathy from osteomyelitis and soft tissue infection? Nucl Med Commun 2007;28:465–72

6.5   Response Assessment

Few studies have tried to explore potential of FDG PET/CT in assessing response to therapy in osteomyelitis. Riccio et al. [21] studied antibiotic treatment response in pyogenic spine infection in 28 patients and concluded that uptake confined to the margins of the destroyed disc should not be considered as persistent infection. However, FDG uptake in bone and/or soft tissue on follow-up was suggestive of poor clinical response. Thus, pattern of uptake along with quantification of metabolic activity was found to be important in assessing response. Treatment response in spondylodiscitis has also been explored. Nanni et al. [22] showed the feasibility and superiority of using changes in SUVmax, as compared to C-reactive protein (CRP), in establishing and monitoring response in patients with haematogenous infective spondylodiscitis. They compared scans at 2 and 4 weeks after initial therapy and found significantly lower SUVmax in responders after 4 weeks. However, further studies are warranted to establish the role of FDG PET/CT in this regard.

Conclusion

FDG PET/CT has demonstrated promising results for imaging of osteomyelitis. It is a useful adjunct to MRI in doubtful cases. It surpasses performance of MRI is spinal infections. It significantly adds to established clinical workup of the diabetic foot. Its ability to assess soft tissue, skeletal, vascular, and neurological (Charcot joints) complications in a single examination may make it an important investigational tool in conjunction with MRI, in this potentially dangerous disease. PET-MRI as a modality may evolve in this regard. However, these aspirations need strengthening with larger prospective research studies in future.

Key Points

- FDG PET/CT scores over conventional modalities for accurate delineation of diabetic foot infections due to its superior resolution.

- FDG PET/CT in osteomyelitis of axial and appendicular skeleton has a sensitivity and specificity of more than 90% in most studies.

- FDG PET/CT in patients with suspected spinal infection with and without metallic implants have shown sensitivities well above 90%, and specificity and accuracy are about 90%.

- CT scan or MRI imaging may be difficult to interpret because of the inability to differentiate degenerative changes and infectious spondylodiscitis.

- The diagnostic sensitivity of FDG PET/CT in patients suspected with infectious spondylodiscitis, approach 100% and specificity of 75–100% which surpasses sensitivity of MRIs. FDG PET/CT in equivocal MRI findings may reduce the need for surgical exploration.

- FDG PET is a highly specific imaging modality for the diagnosis of osteomyelitis in the diabetic foot and should be considered to be a useful complementary imaging modality.

References

1. Bleeker-Rovers CP, Vos FJ, Corstens FH, Oyen WJ. Imaging of infectious diseases using [18F] fluorodeoxyglucose PET. Q J Nucl Med Mol Imaging. 2008;52(1):17–29.
2. de Winter F, van de Wiele C, Vogelaers D, de Smet K, Verdonk R, Dierckx RA. Fluorine-18 fluorodeoxyglucose-position emission tomography: a highly accurate imaging modality for the diagnosis of chronic musculoskeletal infections. J Bone Joint Surg Am. 2001;83-A(5):651–60.
3. Hartmann A, Eid K, Dora C, Trentz O, von Schulthess GK, Stumpe KD. Diagnostic value of 18F-FDG PET/CT in trauma patients with suspected chronic osteomyelitis. Eur J Nucl Med Mol Imaging. 2007;34(5):704–14.
4. Termaat MF, Raijmakers PG, Scholten HJ, Bakker FC, Patka P, Haarman HJ. The accuracy of diagnostic imaging for the assessment of chronic osteomyelitis: a systematic review and metaanalysis. J Bone Joint Surg Am. 2005;87(11):2464–71.
5. Hess S, Hansson SH, Pedersen KT, Basu S, Høilund-Carlsen PF. FDG-PET/CT in infectious and inflammatory diseases. PET Clin. 2014;9:497–519.
6. Gemmel F, Rijk PC, Collins JM, Parlevliet T, Stumpe KD, Palestro CJ. Expanding role of 18F-fluoro-D-deoxyglucose PET and PET/CT in spinal infections. Eur Spine J. 2010;19(4):540–51.
7. Demirev A, Weijers R, Geurts J, Mottaghy F, Walenkamp G, Brans B. Comparison of [18 F]FDG PET/CT and MRI in the diagnosis of active osteomyelitis. Skelet Radiol. 2014;43(5):665–72.
8. Vos FJ, Kullberg BJ, Sturm PD, et al. Metastatic infectious disease and clinical outcome in Staphylococcus aureus and Streptococcus species bacteremia. Medicine. 2012;91(2):86–94.
9. Schmitz A, Risse JH, Grunwald F, Gassel F, Biersack HJ, Schmitt O. Fluorine-18 fluorodeoxy-glucose positron emission tomography findings in spondylodiscitis: preliminary results. Eur Spine J. 2001;10(6):534–9.
10. Stumpe KD, Zanetti M, Weishaupt D, Hodler J, Boos N, Von Schulthess GK. FDG positron emission tomography for differentiation of degenerative and infectious endplate abnormalities in the lumbar spine detected on MR imaging. AJR Am J Roentgenol. 2002;179(5):1151–7.
11. Hungenbach S, Delank KS, Dietlein M, Eysel P, Drzezga A, Schmidt MC. 18F-fluorodeoxyglucose uptake pattern in patients with suspected spondylodiscitis. Nucl Med Commun. 2013;34(11):1068–74.
12. Prodromou ML, Ziakas PD, Poulou LS, Karsaliakos P, Thanos L, Mylonakis E. FDG PET is a robust tool for the diagnosis of spondylodiscitis: a meta-analysis of diagnostic data. Clin Nucl Med. 2014;39(4):330–5.
13. Abbott CA, Carrington AL, Ashe H, et al. The North-West Diabetes Foot Care Study: incidence of, and risk factors for, new diabetic foot ulceration in a community-based patient cohort. Diabet Med. 2002;19:377–84. PMID:12027925.
14. Reiber GE, Vileikyte L, Boyko EJ, et al. Causal pathways for incident lower-extremity ulcers in patients with diabetes from two settings. Diabetes Care. 1999;22:157–62.
15. Marcus CD, Ladam-Marcus VJ, Leone J, et al. MR imaging of osteomyelitis and neuropathic osteoarthropathy in the feet of diabetics. Radiographics. 1996;16:1337–48.

16. Dinh MT, Abad CL, Safdar N. Diagnostic accuracy of physical examination and imaging tests for osteomyelitis underlying diabetic foot ulcers: meta-analysis. Clin Infect Dis. 2008;47(4):519–27.
17. Nawaz A, Torigian DA, Siegelman ES, et al. Diagnostic performance of FDG-PET, MRI, and plain film radiography (PFR) for the diagnosis of osteomyelitis in the diabetic foot. Mol Imaging Biol. 2010;12:335–42.
18. Basu S, Chryssikos T, Houseni M, et al. Potential role of FDG-PET in the setting of diabetic neuroosteoarthropathy: can it differentiate uncomplicated Charcot's neuropathy from osteomyelitis and soft tissue infection? Nucl Med Commun. 2007;28:465–72.
19. Basu S, Zhuang H, Alavi A. Imaging of lower extremity artery atherosclerosis in diabetic foot: FDG-PET imaging and histopathological correlates. Clin Nucl Med. 2007;32(7):567–8.
20. Basu S, Shah J, Houseni M, et al. Uptake in the lower extremity arteries in diabetic foot with ischemic complications and neuropathic osteoarthropathy: FDG PET and histopathological correlation. Clin Nucl Med. 2007;33(1):74–80. [Abstracts from the ACNP34th Annual Meeting, February 15-18, 2007, San Antonio, Texas].
21. Riccio SA, Chu AK, Rabin HR, Kloiber R. Fluorodeoxyglucose positron emission tomography/computed tomography interpretation criteria for assessment of antibiotic treatment response in pyogenic spine infection. Can Assoc Radiol J. 2015;66(2):145–52.
22. Nanni C, Boriani L, Salvadori C, et al. FDG PET/CT is useful for the interim evaluation of response to therapy in patients affected by haematogenous spondylodiscitis. Eur J Nucl Med Mol Imaging. 2012;39(10):1538–44.

^{18}F-FDG PET/CT in Infected Vascular Grafts

7

Ashik Amlani and Thomas Wagner

Contents

Vascular graft insertion to treat aortic or peripheral aneurysm and lower limb occlusive disease is now commonplace [1]. A variety of synthetic materials, autologous veins, or a combination of the two can be used as the graft material depending on the anatomical location and clinical circumstance [2]. Although graft-related complications are uncommon, one of the most feared is graft infection and this remains a major surgical challenge [3]. This chapter will discuss the use of ^{18}F-FDG PET/CT in the diagnosis of vascular graft infection.

Vascular graft infection is a relatively rare occurrence (cumulative incidence 1–6% [4]) although it can cause significant morbidity and mortality. Complications of infection include anastomotic bleeding, sepsis, and conduit thrombosis [5, 6]; resultant limb loss and mortality have been reported as up to 70% and 75%, respectively [7].

One of the difficulties of graft infection is that it is often non-specific in presentation and hence challenging to diagnose. Early-onset infection (defined as those occurring within 4 months of insertion) can present with fever, bacteraemia, wound infection, graft dysfunction with thrombosis or anastomotic bleeding, or abdominal discomfort. Blood tests may show an inflammatory response. Late-onset infection (after 4 months) is usually more insidious with patients presenting with complications such as graft erosion, hydronephrosis, or false aneurysm formation. Fever and

A. Amlani (✉)
Department of Radiology, Guy's and St. Thomas' NHS Foundation Trust, London, UK
e-mail: Ashik.amlani@nhs.net

T. Wagner
Department of Nuclear Medicine, Royal Free London NHS Foundation Trust, London, UK
e-mail: thomas.wagner@nhs.net

© Springer International Publishing AG, part of Springer Nature 2018
T. Wagner, S. Basu (eds.), *PET/CT in Infection and Inflammation*,
Clinicians' Guides to Radionuclide Hybrid Imaging,
https://doi.org/10.1007/978-3-319-90412-2_7

an inflammatory response can be absent [8]. Once diagnosed, surgery remains the mainstay of treatment of graft infection [5].

No current gold standard exists for the diagnosis. Clinical, microbiological, and radiological investigations have all proven useful; however, there are no formal diagnostic criteria or pathways [8]. The most commonly employed imaging modality is contrast enhanced computed tomography (CT). Studies suggest it is accurate in diagnosing advanced graft infection but not low-grade infection (sensitivity 55.5%, specificity 100%) [9]. Advanced infection findings on CT include ectopic gas, focal bowel wall thickening, perigraft fluid, perigraft soft tissue, pseudoaneurysm formation, disruption of the aneurysmal wrap, and increased soft tissue between the graft and surrounding wrap [10]. A further advantage of CT is that simultaneous diagnostic or therapeutic intervention (such as needle aspiration) may be carried out [5]. In low-grade infection, the high risk of false-negative results necessitates the use of alternative structural and functional imaging techniques such as magnetic resonance imaging (MRI), ultrasonography, or white blood cell labelled scintigraphy [6]. Radiolabelled white blood cell scintigraphy with ^{111}In or ^{99m}Tc-HMPAO has been used for years to diagnose graft infection and EANM/SNMMI guidelines suggest PET/CT may not offer any significant advantage over it in this circumstance [11]. However, evidence suggests false-positive rates (especially early post-operatively) are high [12, 13]; these may be from haematomas, lymphoceles, sterile pseudoaneurysms, or infections near the graft [14, 15]. Another drawback is the labour-intensive nature of the scan itself and the length of time it takes to obtain a result when compared to PET/CT [15]. Hybrid imaging in the form of ^{18}F-FDG PET/CT has also shown promise as increased glucose metabolism may be detected earlier or in less florid infection compared to CT findings alone [16]; however, no studies have compared PET/CT with radiolabelled white blood cell scintigraphy.

Several papers have been published in the literature suggesting that ^{18}F-FDG PET/CT improves diagnostic accuracy in graft infection. Case reports published as early as 2003 [17–20] have demonstrated the potential of FDG PET/CT. An early prospective feasibility study by Fukuchi et al. [12] in 33 patients with suspected aortic graft infection graded the intensity of FDG uptake on a five-point scale and whether the uptake was focal or diffuse in nature. An intensity of three or four out of five was thought to be positive for infection. They derived a sensitivity of 91% for FDG PET compared to 64% for CT ($p < 0.05$) and a specificity of 64% compared to 86% (not significant). In a second large prospective study of 39 patients [13], PET/CT had a sensitivity of 93%, specificity of 91%, positive predictive value of 88%, and negative predictive value of 96% for the diagnosis of vascular graft infection. Here, focal increased ^{18}F-FDG uptake in the region of a vascular graft with intensity higher than that of surrounding tissue was defined as infection. Low and medium intensity linear uptake was not defined as infection.

In the largest prospective study to date, 76 patients with 96 various prostheses suspected of being infected underwent ^{18}F-FDG PET/CT scanning [6]. The images were again assessed on the basis of FDG uptake (on a three-point scale) subjectively but also semi-quantitatively using regions of interest to derive maximum FDG uptake compared to blood background. When focal as well as heterogeneous FDG uptake was considered positive, sensitivity, specificity, PPV, and NPV values were 98.2%, 75.6%, 84.4%, and 96.9% respectively [6]. Although semi-quantitative analysis proved to be no more accurate than subjective analysis, graft border irregularity on CT was an independent and significant predictor of graft infection.

More recent studies have assessed graft maximum standardised uptake value (SUVmax) and attempted to determine an optimum cut-off between infected and non-infected prosthesis to minimise false-positives and -negatives. Sah et al. [16] suggested an SUVmax cut-off as greater than 3.7 whereas Tokuda et al. [21] suggested greater than 8. The semi-quantitative analysis by Spacek et al. [6] produced an SUVmax cut-off of 1.7.

Figures 7.1 and 7.2 show two examples of intense uptake on FDG PET/CT in infected vascular grafts. Figure 7.3 shows diffuse moderate uptake in a non-infected graft.

There are drawbacks to FDG PET/CT imaging. ¹⁸F-FDG activity can be increased in scar tissue or post-operatively at sites of wound healing [22]. Similarly, a foreign body low-grade inflammatory reaction can be induced by grafts [23]. Other likely sources of false-positives include an infected haematoma or a lymphocele around the site of the graft [16]. Whilst demonstrating high sensitivity, these findings decrease the specificity of FDG PET/CT in accurately identifying graft infection and it is important to differentiate them from true abnormal uptake within the graft. It has been demonstrated these false-positives could be differentiated from infection by assessing the pattern of uptake. Focal or segmental uptake is more likely to represent infection compared to diffuse uptake; in one paper using this as a diagnostic criterion significantly improved specificity and PPV of FDG PET/CT [12]. Similarly, when prostheses with heterogeneous uptake were excluded from analysis, Spacek et al. [6] reported increased sensitivity and specificity. They consider heterogeneous uptake to decrease accuracy and suggest it is an uncertain finding. Difficulty arises when the entirety of the graft is infected and under these circumstances uptake is likely to be diffuse despite infection.

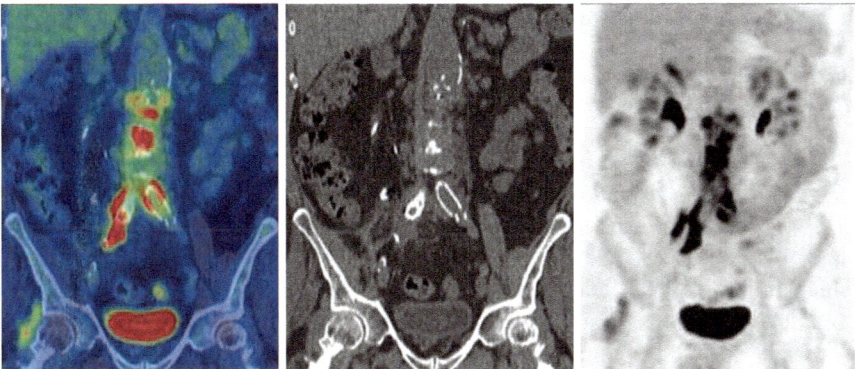

Fig. 7.1 Multifocal intense heterogeneous uptake in the wall of the EVAR and in adjacent soft tissue is very suspicious for infected EVAR

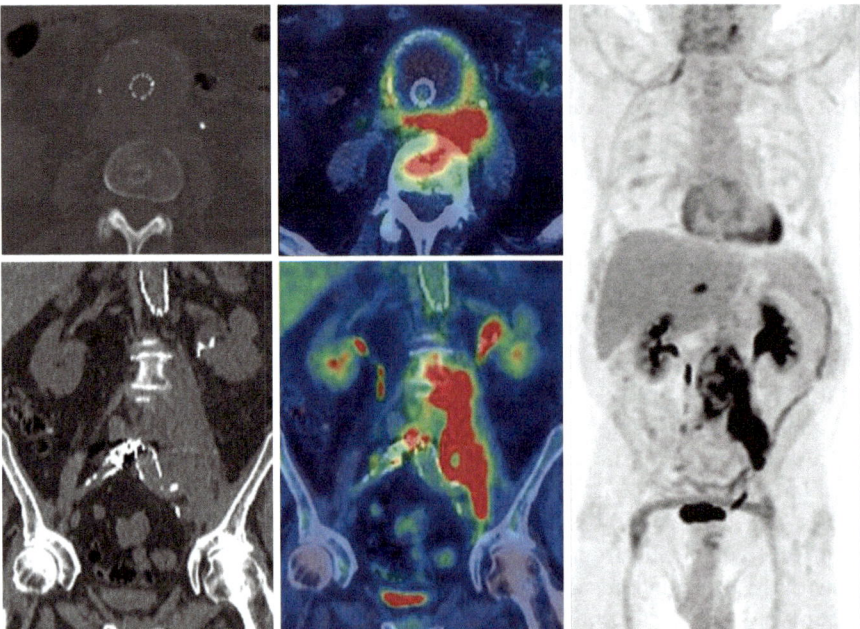

Fig. 7.2 An 82-year-old with a previous EVAR. PUO for the last 4 months, still febrile on wide spectrum triple antibiotic therapy. Intense uptake in soft tissue and wall of the EVAR with abnormal uptake extending into lytic changes in a vertebral body, in keeping with an infected graft

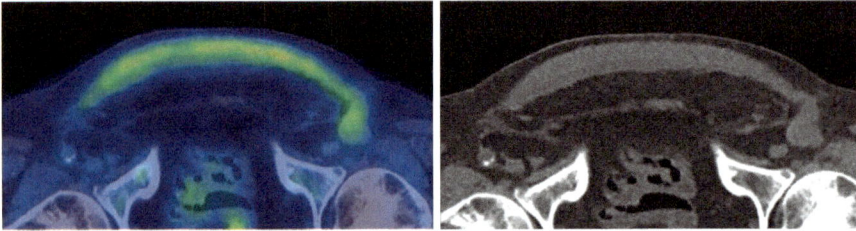

Fig. 7.3 Long-standing diffuse moderate uptake in a femoro-femoral crossover graft, in keeping with benign chronic inflammatory change

Other drawbacks include the lack of a true gold standard with which to compare FDG PET/CT. One study [16] used microorganism detection in perigraft fluid, another [13] used histopathological findings and microbiological assay at surgery whilst a third used positive Gram stain of the prosthesis post-surgery or perigraft fluid [24]. Additionally, study populations varied with, for example, different prior treatment (including antimicrobial therapy) or different graft sites. Whilst most focussed on aortic graft infection, the heterogeneity of the methods and study populations means that drawing comparisons between papers (such as SUVmax values) is difficult. Finally, general drawbacks of PET/CT must be considered.

Of particular relevance here is its relative unavailability out of hours or in an emergency [16].

In conclusion, it is clear that ¹⁸F-FDG PET/CT has the potential to be an extremely valuable modality in the diagnosis of vascular graft infection with high sensitivity. It is likely that a combination of subjective visual grading (in terms of both uptake intensity and pattern) as well as SUVmax cut-off will be used in the future. However, further studies with larger, more homogeneous patient populations must be conducted before SUVmax values can be introduced into clinical practice.

Key Points

- FDG PET/CT is a sensitive non-invasive test to detect infection of vascular grafts. It is complementary to CT angiography. Typical findings in an infected graft are intense focal uptake. Non-infected grafts can demonstrate moderate diffuse smooth uptake for years.

References

1. Swain TW, Calligaro KD, Dougherty MD. Management of infected aortic prosthetic grafts. Vasc Endovasc Surg. 2004;38(1):75–82.
2. Twine CP, McLain AD. Graft type for femoro-popliteal bypass surgery. Cochrane Database Syst Rev. 2010;(5):CD001487.
3. Harris JP. Complications of vascular surgery: infected vascular grafts, aortoenteric fistula, and pseudoaneurysms. General surgery. Springer; 2009. p. 1895–902.
4. Leroy O, Meybeck A, Sarraz-Bournet B, d'Elia P, Legout L. Vascular graft infections. Curr Opin Infect Dis. 2012;25(2):154–8.
5. Perera GB, Fujitani RM, Kubaska SM. Aortic graft infection: update on management and treatment options. Vasc Endovasc Surg. 2006;40(1):1–10.
6. Spacek M, Belohlavek O, Votrubova J, Sebesta P, Stadler P. Diagnostics of "non-acute" vascular prosthesis infection using 18F-FDG PET/CT: our experience with 96 prostheses. Eur J Nucl Med Mol Imaging. 2009;36(5):850–8.
7. Legout L, Sarraz-Bournet B, D'Elia PV, Devos P, Pasquet A, Caillaux M, et al. Characteristics and prognosis in patients with prosthetic vascular graft infection: a prospective observational cohort study. Clin Microbiol Infect. 2012;18(4):352–8.
8. FitzGerald SF, Kelly C, Humphreys H. Diagnosis and treatment of prosthetic aortic graft infections: confusion and inconsistency in the absence of evidence or consensus. J Antimicrob Chemother. 2005;56(6):996–9.
9. Orton DF, LeVeen RF, Saigh JA, Culp WC, Fidler JL, Lynch TJ, et al. Aortic prosthetic graft infections: radiologic manifestations and implications for management. Radiographics. 2000;20(4):977–93.
10. Low RN, Wall SD, Jeffrey RB, Sollitto RA, Reilly LM, Tierney LM. Aortoenteric fistula and perigraft infection: evaluation with CT. Radiology. 1990;175(1):157–62.
11. Jamar F, Buscombe J, Chiti A, Christian PE, Delbeke D, Donohoe KJ, et al. EANM/SNMMI guideline for 18F-FDG use in inflammation and infection. J Nucl Med. 2013;54(4):647–58.
12. Fukuchi K, Ishida Y, Higashi M, Tsunekawa T, Ogino H, Minatoya K, et al. Detection of aortic graft infection by fluorodeoxyglucose positron emission tomography: comparison with computed tomographic findings. J Vasc Surg. 2005;42(5):919–25.

13. Keidar Z, Engel A, Hoffman A, Israel O, Nitecki S. Prosthetic vascular graft infection: the role of 18F-FDG PET/CT. J Nucl Med. 2007;48(8):1230–6.
14. Chung CJ, Wilson AA, Melton JW, Hartley WS, Allen DM. Uptake of In-111 labeled leukocytes by lymphocele. A cause of false-positive vascular graft infection. Clin Nucl Med. 1992;17(5):368–70.
15. Samuel A, Paganelli G, Chiesa R, Sudati F, Calvitto M, Melissano G, et al. Detection of prosthetic vascular graft infection using avidin/indium-111-biotin scintigraphy. J Nucl Med. 1996;37(1):55–61.
16. Sah BR, Husmann L, Mayer D, Scherrer A, Rancic Z, Puippe G, et al. Diagnostic performance of 18F-FDG-PET/CT in vascular graft infections. Eur J Vasc Endovasc Surg. 2015;49(4):455–64.
17. Krupnick AS, Lombardi JV, Engels FH, Kreisel D, Zhuang H, Alavi A, et al. 18-fluorodeoxyglucose positron emission tomography as a novel imaging tool for the diagnosis of aortoenteric fistula and aortic graft infection—a case report. Vasc Endovasc Surg. 2003;37(5):363–6.
18. Shim H, Sung K, Kim WS, Lee YT, Park PW, Jeong DS. Diagnosis of graft infection using FDG PET-CT. Korean J Thorac Cardiovasc Surg. 2012;45(3):189–91.
19. Dutasta F, Richaud C, Michon A, Ragone E, Podglajen I, Mainardi JL. Use of 18F-FDG PET/CT for diagnosis of vascular graft infection with spread to sternum caused by Coxiella burnetii. Infect Dis (Lond). 2016;48(10):769–71.
20. Lauwers P, Van den Broeck S, Carp L, Hendriks J, Van Schil P, Blockx P. The use of positron emission tomography with (18)F-fluorodeoxyglucose for the diagnosis of vascular graft infection. Angiology. 2007;58(6):717–24.
21. Tokuda Y, Oshima H, Araki Y, Narita Y, Mutsuga M, Kato K, et al. Detection of thoracic aortic prosthetic graft infection with 18F-fluorodeoxyglucose positron emission tomography/computed tomography. Eur J Cardiothorac Surg. 2013;43(6):1183–7.
22. Cook GJR, Fogelman I, Maisey MN. Normal physiological and benign pathological variants of 18-fluoro-2-deoxyglucose positron-emission tomography scanning: potential for error in interpretation. Semin Nucl Med. 1996;26(4):308–14.
23. Keidar Z, Pirmisashvili N, Leiderman M, Nitecki S, Israel O. 18F-FDG uptake in noninfected prosthetic vascular grafts: incidence, patterns, and changes over time. J Nucl Med. 2014;55(3):392–5.
24. Bruggink JL, Glaudemans AW, Saleem BR, Meerwaldt R, Alkefaji H, Prins TR, et al. Accuracy of FDG-PET-CT in the diagnostic work-up of vascular prosthetic graft infection. Eur J Vasc Endovasc Surg. 2010;40(3):348–54.

PET and Cardiac Infections

8

Deborah Pencharz

Contents

A range of organisms including viral, bacterial, and fungal can infect the endocardium, cardiac prosthetic devices, pericardium, and myocardium. Currently, most evidence on the use of FDG PET/CT regards its use in prosthetic cardiac components and valves. It should also be noted that echocardiography, CT, and MRI play a useful role in the investigation of potential or proven cardiac infections. A good overview of these modalities, together with helpful descriptions of the pathophysiology of cardiac infections, has been described in a recent review article [1].

D. Pencharz
Department of Nuclear Medicine, Brighton and Sussex University Hospitals NHS Trust,
Royal Sussex County Hospital, Brighton, UK
e-mail: Deborah.pencharz@bsuh.nhs.uk

© Springer International Publishing AG, part of Springer Nature 2018   71
T. Wagner, S. Basu (eds.), *PET/CT in Infection and Inflammation*,
Clinicians' Guides to Radionuclide Hybrid Imaging,
https://doi.org/10.1007/978-3-319-90412-2_8

8.1   Preparation for Cardiac PET/CT

Normal myocardium has variable uptake of glucose and the standard 4–6 h fast prior to a PET/CT does not consistently suppress physiological cardiac FDG uptake to allow accurate evaluation of pathological uptake. However, the combination of a high fat, low carbohydrate diet followed by prolonged fasting (e.g. 18 h) as been shown to significantly suppress physiological uptake [2–4]. Protocols using this type of preparation are required when assessing for cardiac infections. The use of unfractionated heparin to further supress myocardial uptake has also been described [5] and is used in some centres [6].

8.2   Native Valve Infective Endocarditis

FDG PET/CT is not typically used for the diagnosis of native valve infectious endocarditis (IE), diagnosis is based on the modified Duke criteria which includes clinical, echocardiographic, and biological findings, as well as the results of blood cultures and serology [7]. Recent European Society of Cardiology (ESC) guidelines on endocarditis [8] have maintained this approach and have also provided further modified diagnostic criteria.

The rationale for this is due to the published low sensitivity of FDG PET/CT in detecting native valve IE. A recent systematic review and meta-analysis [9] demonstrated a sensitivity of 61%, lower than the modified Duke criteria of 80% [8]. Additionally, a recent cross-sectional study found that PET/CT was false-negative in all cases of suspected native valve IE ($n = 21$) [6].

However, FDG PET/CT has proved to be useful in detecting septic emboli in patients with native valve IE. In a prospective cohort study of patients with definite IE, the systematic use of PET/CT in 47 patients compared to 94 controls who did not have IE showed that PET/CT diagnosed significantly more infectious complications (septic emboli) (18% vs. 57.4%, $p = 0.0001$) and was associated with a two-fold reduction in the number of relapses (9.6% vs. 4.2%, $p = 0.25$) [10]. The ESC guidelines [8] have included imaging for embolic events, which can be performed with FDG PET/CT, in the further diagnostic workup of patients who fall into the "possible" category of the modified Duke criteria.

8.3   Prosthetic Valve Endocarditis

Diagnosis of prosthetic valve IE (PVE) is more challenging than native valve IE due to more atypical presentation and more frequently negative blood cultures and echocardiography [8]. The use of PET/CT in the evaluation of patients with possible PVE, according to Duke criteria, is now recommended in recently published ESC guidelines on IE [8]. In these guidelines, abnormal activity around the site of implantation detected by ^{18}F-FDG PET/CT (if the prosthesis was implanted >3 months previously) is considered a major criterion. This is based on a study of FDG PET/CT in PVE which found a sensitivity, specificity, positive predictive value, negative predictive value, and accuracy of 73% (95% CI: 54–87%), 80% (56–93%), 85% (64–95%), 67% (45–84%), and 76% (63–86%), respectively. Use of FDG PET/CT increased the sensitivity of the modified Duke's criteria at admission from 70% (52–83%) to 97% (83–99%), $p = 0.008$ [11].

8.4   Cardiac Implantable Electronic Device Infections

Cardiac implantable electronic devices (CIED) include pacemakers and implantable cardioverter defibrillators. When considering infections of these devices, it is important to be aware of the distinction between an infection limited to the generator pocket versus an infection extending to the cardiac leads, valves, or endocardium although differentiating between the two types of infection can be difficult.

Similarly to PVE, diagnosis can be challenging. Echocardiography plays a lead role in the diagnosis of CIED infection; however, a normal echo does not rule it out. There is increasing evidence of the usefulness of FDG PET/CT in suspected CIED infection. The recent ESC guidelines [8] state: *"Radiolabelled leucocyte scintigraphy and ^{18}F-FDG PET/CT scanning may be considered additive tools in patients with suspected cardiac device related IE, positive blood cultures and negative echocardiography"*. In addition, recent evidence-based guidelines on the use of PET/CT in the United Kingdom [12] state PET/CT is indicated in the "evaluation of… cardiac implantable device related infection in selected cases provided sufficient time has elapsed since surgery".

These recommendations are based on a number of studies. One study [13] compared three groups of patients: group A consisted of 42 patients with suspected CIED infection, group B included 12 patients without infection who underwent PET/CT 4–8 weeks post-implant and group C included 12 patients implanted for >6 months without infection who underwent PET/CT for another indication. A ratio between maximal suspicious cardiac uptake and lung parenchymal uptake (cardiac$_{max}$:lung$_{mean}$) was calculated. In Group A, 32 patients had positive PET/CT, 24 of these underwent extraction with excellent correlation. In 7 patients with positive PET/CT, 6 were treated as superficial infection with clinical resolution. One patient with positive PET/CT but negative leukocyte scan was considered false positive due to a Dacron pouch. Ten patients with negative-PET/CT were treated with antibiotics and none had relapsed at 12.9 ± 1.9 months. Group B patients had mild uptake seen at the level of the connector, group C patients did not demonstrate any abnormal uptake. Median cardiac$_{max}$:lung$_{mean}$ was significantly higher in Group A (2.02) vs. B (1.08) vs. C (0.57); $p < 0.001$.

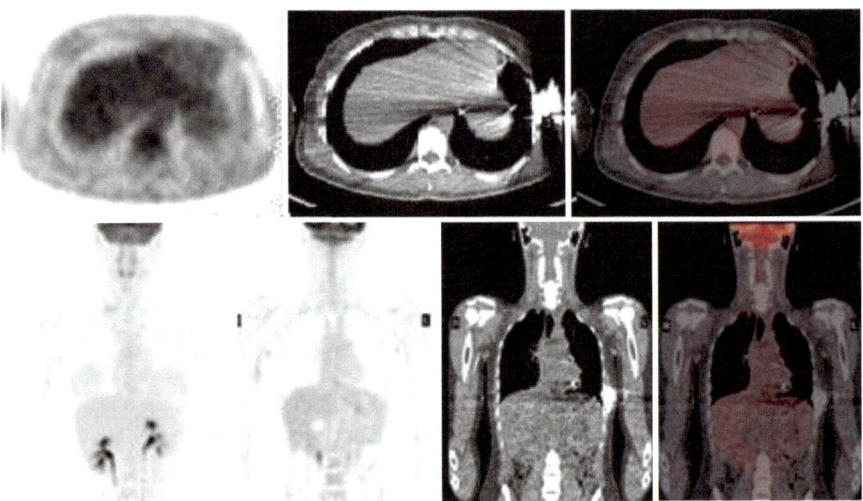

Fig. 8.1 No CIED infection. There is no uptake in the device pocket or lead to suggest infection. Most modern PET /CT scanners have provisions for metal artefact reduction allowing accurate assessment of metabolic activity

A later study used similar methods to analyse the use of FDG PET/CT to detect pocket infection in CIEDs [14]. It used a ratio of maximum count rate around the CIED to mean normal lung parenchymal count rate ($pocket_{max}:lung_{mean}$) in patients with and without (controls) suspected CIED pocket infection, patients were managed independently of PET/CT result. Patients with suspected generator pocket infection that required CIED extraction ($n = 32$) had significantly higher ^{18}F-FDG activity compared with those that did not require extraction ($n = 14$) or controls ($n = 40$). The $pocket_{max}:lung_{mean}$ was: 4.80 (3.18–7.05) vs. 1.40 (0.88–1.73) vs. 1.10 (0.98–1.40), respectively; $p < 0.001$. The area under the receiver operator characteristic analysis for the $pocket_{max}:lung_{mean}$ was 0.98 for those ultimately needing extraction with an optimal cut-off value of >2.0 (sensitivity 97%, specificity 98%).

A smaller study consisted of 27 patients [15] with suspected CIED infection who had an initial PET/CT and a final diagnosis made via culture in those who had leads removed or clinical/instrumental follow-up after 6 months in those who did not. Among the ten patients with a positive PET/CT scan, seven received a final diagnosis of "definite IE", one of "possible IE", and two of "IE rejected". Among the 17 patients with a negative-PET/CT scan, four were false-negative and received a final diagnosis of definite IE. These patients underwent PET/CT after having started antibiotic therapy (≥48 h) or had a technically suboptimal examination.

Figure 8.1 shows an example of a non-infected CIED. Figure 8.2 shows increased uptake in an infected prosthetic aortic valve prosthesis. Figure 8.3 shows infection of a device pocket with extension to the lead.

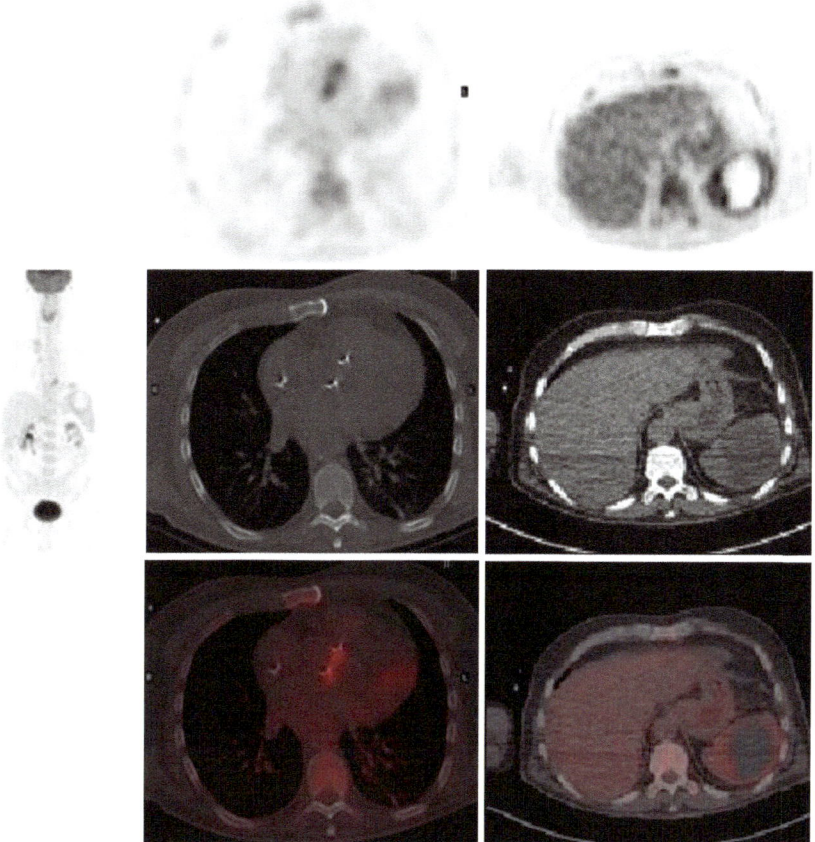

Fig. 8.2 Aortic valve endocarditis with splenic abscess. There is focal uptake in the prosthetic aortic valve suggesting infective endocarditis. There is a large photopaenic area in the spleen with a rim of metabolic activity suggesting abscess. Whole body imaging allows evaluation of ectopic source of infection

8.5   Pericarditis

It is important to remember there are mulitple non-infectious causes of pericarditis, some of the most common being autoimmune and malignant (particularly lung, breast, and lymphoma) [16] and PET/CT is frequently used in investigating these pathologies. Viruses are the most common cause of pericarditis in the developed world and TB in the developing world [16].

ESC guidelines on pericarditis are not specific on the use of PET/CT stating [16]: "PET/CT can be indicated to depict the metabolic activity of pericardial disease" (p. 2942). However, the guidelines do further elaborate that it is useful in

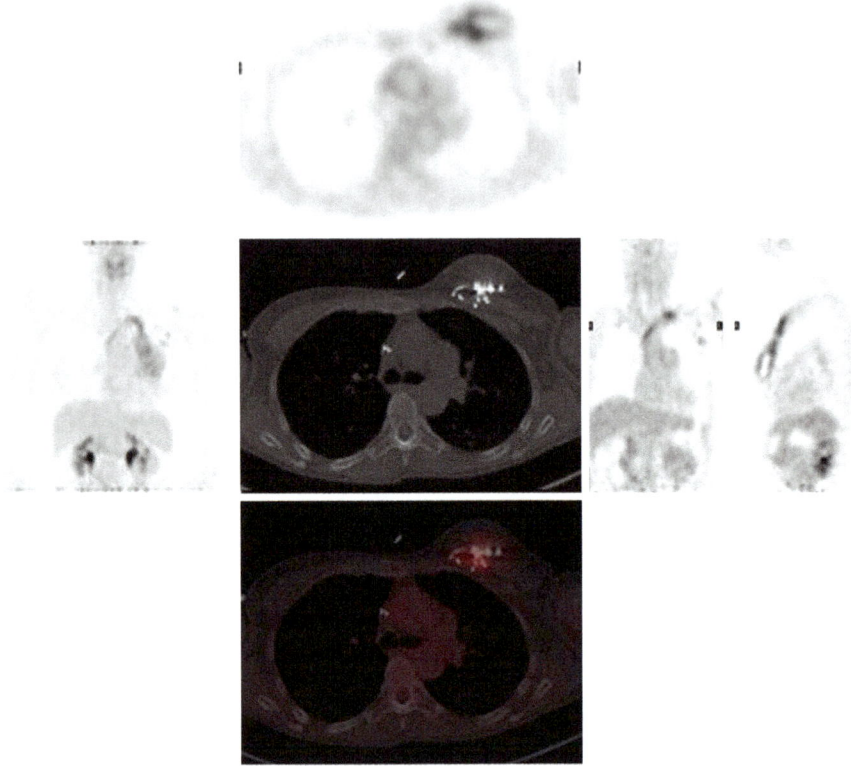

Fig. 8.3 Device pocket infection with extension to the lead. There is uptake in the device pocket with tracer uptake tracking along the intravascular part of the lead stopping short of the intra cardiac insertion

distinguishing TB from idiopathic pericarditis, this is based on a study of 15 patients which retrospectively evaluated the ability of PET/CT to distingish between the two aetiologies [17]. This found that the mean and standard deviation (SD) of pericardial thickness and SUVmax of acute tuberculous pericarditis was significantly higher than in acute idiopathic pericarditis (5.1 SD [1.0] vs. 3.4 [0.9], $p < 0.05$; 13.5 [3.9] vs. 3.0 [0.7], $p < 0.05$, respectively). The mean and SD SUVmax of mediastinal and supraclavicular lymph nodes of acute tuberculous pericarditis (5.3 [1.8]) was significantly higher than that of acute idiopathic pericarditis (2.8 [0.6], $p < 0.05$). There was no significant difference in the mean size of the mediastinal and supraclavicular lymph nodes between acute tuberculous and idiopathic pericarditis.

8.6   Myocarditis

A variety of infectious and systemic diseases can also cause myocarditis. Viruses, often enteroviruses, are the most important causes in developed countries [18, 19]. Electrocardiogram, myocardiocytolysis markers, and transthoracic echocardiography are the standard first-line investigations, cardiac MRI is useful to provide further structural and functional information and endomyocardial biopsy is the gold standard diagnostic test [19].

ESC guidelines state (p. 2642) [19]: "Nuclear imaging is not routinely recommended in the diagnosis of myocarditis, with the possible exception of suspected cardiac sarcoidosis" and a relatively recent review on FDG PET in cardiac infections also does not describe any specific role for PET/CT [18]

Conclusion

- There are recommedations and evidence that FDG PET/CT is of use in evaluating patients with suspected prosthetic valve or CIED infection when initial investigations/diagnostic criteria are inconclusive.
- $cardiac_{max}:lung_{mean}$ or $pocket_{max}:lung_{mean}$ has been shown to be a useful parameter when assessing for CIED infection.
- FDG PET/CT should not currently be used to directly investigate for native valve IE. However, in suspected native valve endocarditis, it can be used to look for septic emboli, the knoweldge of which is useful when managing patients with suspected IE.
- FDG PET is currently not routinely used to assess patients with pericarditis or myocarditis; however, it has been shown to help distinguish between idiopathic and TB pericarditis.

Key Points

- There are recommendations and evidence that FDG PET/CT is of use in evaluating patients with suspected prosthetic valve or CIED infection when initial investigations/diagnostic criteria are inconclusive.

- FDG PET/CT should not currently be used to directly investigate for native valve IE. However, in suspected native valve endocarditis, it can be used to look for septic emboli, the knowledge of which is useful when managing patients with suspected IE.

- FDG PET is currently not routinely used to assess patients with pericarditis or myocarditis however it has been shown to help distinguish between idiopathic and TB pericarditis.

References

1. Murillo H, Restrepo CS, Marmol-Velez JA, Vargas D, Ocazionez D, Martinez-Jimenez S, et al. Infectious diseases of the heart: pathophysiology, clinical and imaging overview. Radiographics. 2016;36(4):963–83.
2. Harisankar CN, Mittal BR, Agrawal KL, Abrar ML, Bhattacharya A. Utility of high fat and low carbohydrate diet in suppressing myocardial FDG uptake. J Nucl Cardiol. 2011;18(5):926–36.

3. Williams G, Kolodny GM. Suppression of myocardial 18F-FDG uptake by preparing patients with a high-fat, low-carbohydrate diet. AJR Am J Roentgenol. 2008;190(2):W151–6.
4. Lum DP, Wandell S, Ko J, Coel MN. Reduction of myocardial 2-deoxy-2-[18F]fluoro-D-glucose uptake artifacts in positron emission tomography using dietary carbohydrate restriction. Mol Imaging Biol. 2002;4(3):232–7.
5. Scholtens AM, Verberne HJ, Budde RP, Lam MG. Additional heparin preadministration improves cardiac glucose metabolism suppression over low-carbohydrate diet alone in ^{18}F-FDG PET imaging. J Nucl Med. 2016;57(4):568–73.
6. Granados U, Fuster D, Pericas JM, Llopis J, Ninot S, Quintana E, et al. Diagnostic accuracy of 18F-FDG PET/CT in infective endocarditis and implantable cardiac electronic device infection: a cross-sectional study. J Nucl Med. 2016;57(11):1726–32.
7. Li JS, Sexton DJ, Mick N, Nettles R, Fowler VG Jr, Ryan T, et al. Proposed modifications to the Duke criteria for the diagnosis of infective endocarditis. Clin Infect Dis. 2000;30(4):633–8.
8. The 2015 ESC guidelines for the management of infective endocarditis. Eur Heart J. 2015;36(44):3036–7.
9. Yan J, Zhang C, Niu Y, Yuan R, Zeng X, Ge X, et al. The role of 18F-FDG PET/CT in infectious endocarditis: a systematic review and meta-analysis. Int J Clin Pharmacol Ther. 2016;54(5):337–42.
10. Kestler M, Munoz P, Rodriguez-Creixems M, Rotger A, Jimenez-Requena F, Mari A, et al. Role of (18)F-FDG PET in patients with infectious endocarditis. J Nucl Med. 2014;55(7):1093–8.
11. Saby L, Laas O, Habib G, Cammilleri S, Mancini J, Tessonnier L, et al. Positron emission tomography/computed tomography for diagnosis of prosthetic valve endocarditis: increased valvular 18F-fluorodeoxyglucose uptake as a novel major criterion. J Am Coll Cardiol. 2013;61(23):2374–82.
12. Scarsbrook A, Barrington S. Evidence based indications for the use of PET-CT in the United Kingdom 2016. https://www.rcr.ac.uk/sites/default/files/publication/bfcr163_pet-ct.pdf.
13. Sarrazin JF, Philippon F, Tessier M, Guimond J, Molin F, Champagne J, et al. Usefulness of fluorine-18 positron emission tomography/computed tomography for identification of cardiovascular implantable electronic device infections. J Am Coll Cardiol. 2012;59(18):1616–25.
14. Ahmed FZ, James J, Cunnington C, Motwani M, Fullwood C, Hooper J, et al. Early diagnosis of cardiac implantable electronic device generator pocket infection using (1)(8)F-FDG-PET/CT. Eur Heart J Cardiovasc Imaging. 2015;16(5):521–30.
15. Graziosi M, Nanni C, Lorenzini M, Diemberger I, Bonfiglioli R, Pasquale F, et al. Role of (1)(8)F-FDG PET/CT in the diagnosis of infective endocarditis in patients with an implanted cardiac device: a prospective study. Eur J Nucl Med Mol Imaging. 2014;41(8):1617–23.
16. Adler Y, Charron P, Imazio M, Badano L, Baron-Esquivias G, Bogaert J, et al. 2015 ESC guidelines for the diagnosis and management of pericardial diseases: the Task Force for the Diagnosis and Management of Pericardial Diseases of the European Society of Cardiology (ESC)Endorsed by: The European Association for Cardio-Thoracic Surgery (EACTS). Eur Heart J. 2015;36(42):2921–64.
17. Dong A, Dong H, Wang Y, Cheng C, Zuo C, Lu J. (18)F-FDG PET/CT in differentiating acute tuberculous from idiopathic pericarditis: preliminary study. Clin Nucl Med. 2013;38(4):e160–5.
18. Erba PA, Sollini M, Lazzeri E, Mariani G. FDG-PET in cardiac infections. Semin Nucl Med. 2013;43(5):377–95.
19. Caforio AL, Pankuweit S, Arbustini E, Basso C, Gimeno-Blanes J, Felix SB, et al. Current state of knowledge on aetiology, diagnosis, management, and therapy of myocarditis: a position statement of the European Society of Cardiology Working Group on Myocardial and Pericardial Diseases. Eur Heart J. 2013;34(33):2636–48, 48a–48d.

FDG PET/CT in Autoimmune Diseases

9

Alok Pawaskar and Sandip Basu

Contents

9.1 Introduction

Systemic autoimmune diseases are a heterogeneous group of disorders in which "self-tolerance" has been overcome by genetic and environmental factors and an immune response has been mounted against the body's own organs, tissues, and

A. Pawaskar
Radiation Medicine Centre, Bhabha Atomic Research Centre, Tata Memorial Centre Annexe, Mumbai, India

HCG Manavata Cancer Centre, Nashik, India

S. Basu (✉)
Radiation Medicine Centre, Bhabha Atomic Research Centre, Tata Memorial Centre Annexe, Mumbai, India

Homi Bhabha National Institute, Mumbai, India

© Springer International Publishing AG, part of Springer Nature 2018
T. Wagner, S. Basu (eds.), *PET/CT in Infection and Inflammation*,
Clinicians' Guides to Radionuclide Hybrid Imaging,
https://doi.org/10.1007/978-3-319-90412-2_9

cells [1]. Diagnosis and treatment monitoring of these diseases is primarily done by clinical evaluation, inflammatory markers and biopsy wherever feasible. Role of anatomical imaging is limited to demonstrating tissue or organ destruction caused by the autoimmune processes. Functional imaging, on the other hand, can show the actual process of inflammation caused by activated immune cells in the target organ. Traditionally ^{99m}Tc-colloid, radiolabelled immunoglobulins, bone scan, Gallium-67 scan have been used for this purpose. FDG PET/CT has been extensively used as research tool in autoimmune disorders (AID).

The conventional Nuclear Medicine techniques are time consuming, lack both sensitivity and specificity apart from having low resolution and two-dimensional imaging capabilities. FDG PET/CT on the other hand directly visualizes abnormally increased glucose metabolism in the activated immune cells at the site of inflammation. It has high resolution and target-to-background ratio leading to better sensitivity. The CT component of PET/CT adds to the specificity and exact anatomical localization. Whole body FDG PET/CT imaging can be undertaken in reasonably short time with visualization of complete disease extent in the body. Although biopsy remains gold standard for diagnosis, PET/CT scan can show most accessible site for biopsy and help in diagnosis, where biopsy site is inaccessible. Individuals with autoimmune diseases have increased susceptibility for developing malignancy [2, 3]. FDG PET/CT can potentially image those malignancies in the same scan. One important advantage of FDG PET/CT is ability to quantify metabolic activity at the site of inflammation which makes serial monitoring of response to therapy possible. In this communication, we shall explore the role of FDG PET/CT in individual autoimmune diseases based upon peer-reviewed literature on the subject.

9.2   Autoimmune Vasculitis

It is an inflammatory disease characterized by inflammation and necrosis in the vessel wall leading to reactive destruction of blood vessels. Histopathological analysis is considered as the gold standard for the diagnosis. FDG PET/CT can help in accurate localization of biopsy site and in case the biopsy site is inaccessible, PET/CT can still confirm the diagnosis. Being whole body imaging, it helps to evaluate disease extent. It appears the best choice for early diagnosis and treatment monitoring: CT, MRI, or USG are not useful in early stages due to subtle morphologic changes, or for response assessment due to slow changes. FDG PET/CT is very useful for evaluation of vasculitis in big- or medium-sized vessels, whereas small vessel vasculitis is below the detection limit of current PET/CT scanners. Polymyalgia rheumatica with giant cell arteritis is the most common vasculitis entity affecting medium and large vessels. Significant number of patients also have extra-cranial disease manifestations at the time of diagnosis; especially aortic involvement has a very serious implication such as aortic dissection; hence, the reliable evaluation of it is of critical importance.

Bleeker-Rovers et al. [4] for the first time showed FDG PET to be a useful imaging technique in diagnosing and determining the extent of vasculitis. After this, a number of studies have been done and FDG PET has been shown to have sensitivities of 77–92% and specificities of 89–100% in treatment-naïve patients [5]. FDG PET/CT is able to locate more vascular sites involved than MRI, but they were found to be equivalent in making the initial diagnosis [6]. The treatment of vasculitis reduces the FDG uptake in the vessels thereby lowering the sensitivity in post-treatment patients. However, this property can be used to evaluate treatment response [7]. As compared to anatomical imaging modalities, FDG PET is probably better to predict early response to therapy since morphological changes develop later than the metabolic response.

In a systematic review, Treglia et al. [8] evaluated 32 studies including more than 600 patients and concluded that FDG PET/CT is useful in the initial diagnosis, assessment of activity, and extent of disease in patients with large vessel vasculitis. The review also highlighted the role of FDG PET/CT in assessing disease activity under immuno-suppressive treatment, in predicting relapse, or in evaluating vascular complications. They suggested need for standardization of the techniques employed regarding PET analysis and diagnostic criteria.

9.3   Systemic Lupus Erythematosus (SLE), Polyarteritis Nodosa, and Wegener's Granulomatosis

These autoimmune diseases preferentially involve small- to medium-sized arteries. There are few reports of FDG PET used to study CNS involvement in patients with Wegener's granulomatosis [9] and polyarteritis nodosa [10]. These studies highlight potential role of FDG PET/CT in autoimmune-mediated CNS diseases. In the initial studies of FDG PET for detecting CNS involvement in patients with SLE, glucose metabolism was found to be reduced during active focal and diffuse disease [11]. In these and the subsequent studies, FDG PET was considered to be the most sensitive method for demonstrating reversible deficits and for correlating the functional imaging results with neurological findings.

9.4   Inflammatory Bowel Disease

Chronic inflammatory bowel disease (IBD) includes Crohn's Disease (CD) and ulcerative colitis (UC). These diseases need monitoring of disease activity and disease extent. Currently, there are scoring systems requiring multiple invasive endoscopies (e.g., gastroscopy, colonoscopy, capsule endoscopy) and imaging studies submitting the patients to high doses of radiation (e.g., SBFT, CT, enteroclysis). FDG PET/CT being accurate and non-invasive imaging method for inflammation imaging is likely to be significantly better for the management of these patients.

The first study with stand-alone PET published in 1997 by Bicik et al. [12] used FDG PET in seven patients with suspected IBD, and they found high FDG activity in areas of active inflammation on biopsy and generally higher FDG uptake in patients with clinically active disease. Neurath et al. [13] used FDG PET in patients with known IBD to assess disease extent and found PET to be much more sensitive (85%) than MRI (41%) with comparable specificity. A meta-analysis by Treglia et al. found an overall pooled per segment sensitivity and specificity of 85% and 87%, respectively, reported by various studies [14]. Role of FDG PET in detecting and differentiating fibrostenosis (requiring surgery) versus inflammatory strictures requiring only conservative medical treatment was studied by some [15, 16]. Spier BJ studied use of FDG PET/CT for assessment of response to treatment with implications for treatment strategy [17].

IBD pose a diagnostic challenge in children and adolescence because of invasive endoscopies in them requiring general anesthesia. Hence, non-invasive imaging like FDG PET/CT would be a much preferred option. In a review of literature by Malham M et al. [18], from 1999 to 2013 results were encouraging with a potential for detecting gastrointestinal inflammation with high sensitivity and reasonable specificity. Moreover, the ability of PET/CT to visualize the extraintestinal manifestations of IBD has proven valuable in the diagnostic workup of adults and the same may be expected in a pediatric setting [19]. Hence, although literature is limited, FDG PET/CT has promising potential in IBD in adult and more so in pediatric population.

9.5   Psoriasis and Rheumatoid Arthritis

Psoriasis is chronic autoimmune inflammatory condition typically affecting the skin, but it is also often associated with an inflammatory arthritis - psoriatic arthritis (PsA). In 2001, Yun et al. described the first reported case of increased FDG uptake on a PET scan in joints with active PsA [20]. Takata et al. showed that FDG PET/CT can visualize arthritic joints and entheses in psoriasis patients. Moreover, they showed that PET can be used to asses efficacy of treatment with tumor necrosis factor-α (TNF-α) inhibitors on symptomatic and asymptomatic PsA as well [21].

Rheumatoid arthritis (RA) is another autoimmune condition characterized by symmetric/asymmetrical joint involvement with synovial inflammation, which in advanced stages leads to irreversible destruction of joints due to formation of pannus and cartilage erosion. In a systematic review of FDG PET imaging in joint disorders comprising RA; Carey et al. [22] highlighted the importance of detecting RA, specifically the synovial inflammation as early as possible to arrest progression to advanced stages. FDG PET being whole body imaging seems to be highly useful in assessing global disease activity and/or inflammation burden. Beckers et al. suggested that the degree of FDG uptake may be an indirect measure of neovascularization and consequently aggressive synovitis [23], thereby possibly predicting the course of newly detected, early RA. It is stated that high FDG uptake in large joints is correlated with the risk of developing atlantoaxial instability, a possibly severely debilitating condition. Few studies have shown that FDG PET/CT may be able to predict the outcome of instituted treatment with both traditional treatment (steroids and disease-modifying antirheumatic drugs) [24] and biological treatment (tumor necrosis factor α-inhibitors, TNF-α-inhibitors) [25]. The newer quantification parameters are of important value in treatment response assessment in rheumatoid arthritis with FDG PET/CT [26, 27] (Figs. 9.1 and 9.2) the inflammation in both psoriasis and RA is systemic in nature, and FDG PET/CT has been used to illustrate inflammation in not only skin lesions in psoriasis and joints, but also in the large blood vessels in both psoriasis and RA [28–31] as well as other extra-articular foci of inflammation including regional lymph nodes.

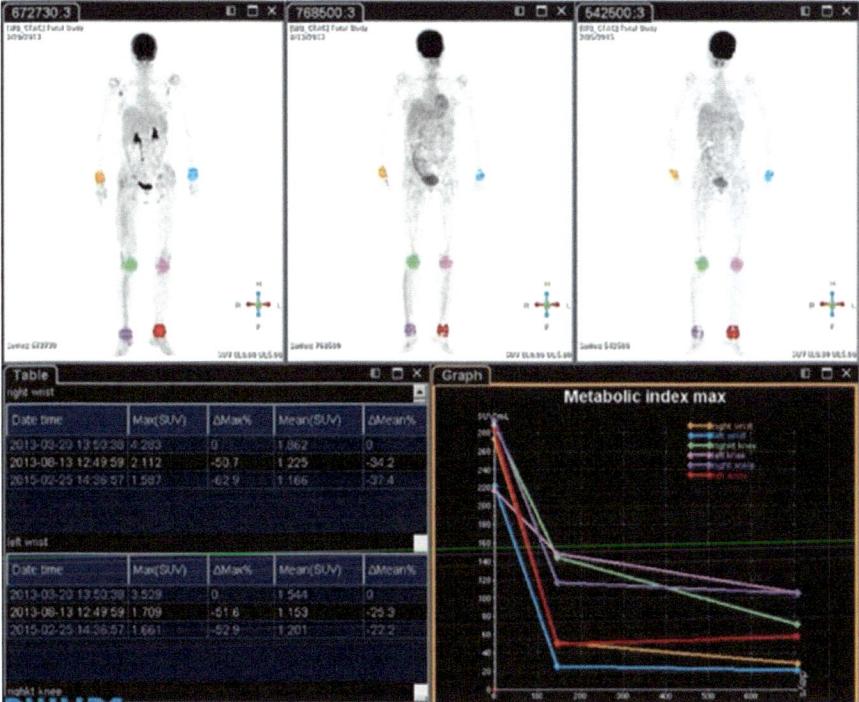

Fig. 9.1 The fluoro-2-deoxy-ᴅ-glucose-positron emission tomography/computed tomography scan showing overall good response. The upper three images are the maximum intensity projection images (at baseline, 3, and 6 months from left to right) showing the joint involvement and extra-articular lesions including bilateral axillary nodes and inguinal nodes at baseline study. There is a good response noted in the joints in the subsequent follow-ups. The lymph nodes also showed a significant response with no uptake in the follow-up scans. The metabolic volumetric product response (in the form of metabolic index max) response is depicted graphically as shown by the curves (Reproduced with permission from Kumar et al. [26])

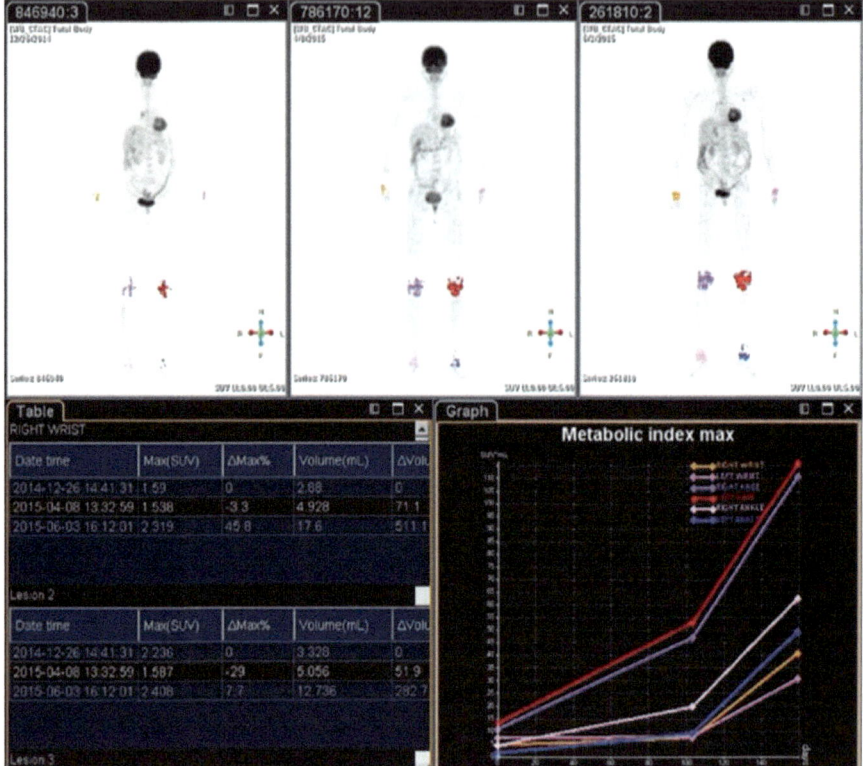

Fig. 9.2 Fluoro-2-deoxy-D-glucose-positron emission tomography/computed tomography show-ing overall no response to both first-line and step-up therapy. The upper three images are maximum intensity projection images showing the joint involvement at baseline, 3, and 6 months. There is an increase in the active inflammation noted in the joints in the first follow-up which is also illustrated by the rise in the curve. This patient was advised etoricoxib, hydroxychloroquine after the baseline scan. After the first follow-up, a step-up therapy was used with addition of methotrexate. The sub-sequent scan also showed no response with increasing activity. The response is depicted graphi-cally as shown by the rising curves for metabolic volumetric product (Reproduced with permission from Kumar et al. [26])

9.6   Autoimmune Brain Diseases

Multiple sclerosis (MS) is an immune-mediated inflammatory, demyelinating disease of the CNS. FDG PET can reveal the localization and distribution of cerebral hypometabolism in relation to demyelinating lesions in the white matter and as well as change in glucose metabolism of cortex, basal ganglia, and cerebellum [32]. FDG PET/CT is also useful in MS patients with cognitive dysfunction for investigation of global and regional cerebral glucose metabolism in comparison to MRI findings [33]. According to Bakshi et al. [34] and Derache et al. [35], FDG PET scans have clinical application as a marker for assessment of disease activity and response to immunotherapy. Autoimmune cerebellar ataxia may be caused by auto-antibodies to various cerebellar targets. Certain investigations reveal a reduction in absolute values of regional cerebral glucose metabolism in the cerebellar hemispheres and vermis, as well as in the brainstem or dentate nuclei [36, 37].

Autoimmune limbic encephalitis is a severe, neuropsychiatric disorder that affects the limbic system, which is responsible for the basic autonomic functions. Autoimmune limbic encephalitis (ALE) may be either paraneoplastic, which is associated with a large number of cancers (lung, breast, testicular, thymoma, Hodgkin's lymphoma) or idiopathic (non-paraneoplastic). According to Fisher et al. [38], PET/CT findings are specific to the disease and have a combination of pronounced occipital hypometabolism and hypermetabolism in the temporal and orbitofrontal cortex. Rey et al. [39] reported three cases with non-paraneoplastic limbic encephalitis characterized by FDG PET bilateral striatal hypermetabolism, in contrast to diffuse hypometabolism in the rest of the brain.

9.7 Sjögren's Disease, Autoimmune Pancreatitis, and Thyroiditis

The list of autoimmune disorders and role of FDG PET/CT in this entity has continuously increasing. Like Shih et al. have described it in case of Sjögren's disease [40]; Nakajo have described role of PET/CT in autoimmune pancreatitis associated with extrapancreatic autoimmune disease [41]. Yoon Lee et al. concluded that in difficult cases, the presence of diffuse uptake of FDG by the pancreas or concomitant extrapancreatic uptake by the salivary glands can be used to aid in differentiation of autoimmune pancreatitis and pancreatic cancer [42]. Although not primarily used for diagnosis, diffuse increased FDG uptake seen in both lobes of thyroid gland is often associated with autoimmune thyroiditis [43].

Immunoglobulin G4-related systemic disease is another important autoimmune disorder, where FDG PET/CT has aided in assessing the extent of the disease, locate the best site for biopsy, and also evaluate the response to treatment and diagnose the suspicion of recurrence [44–46] (Fig. 9.3).

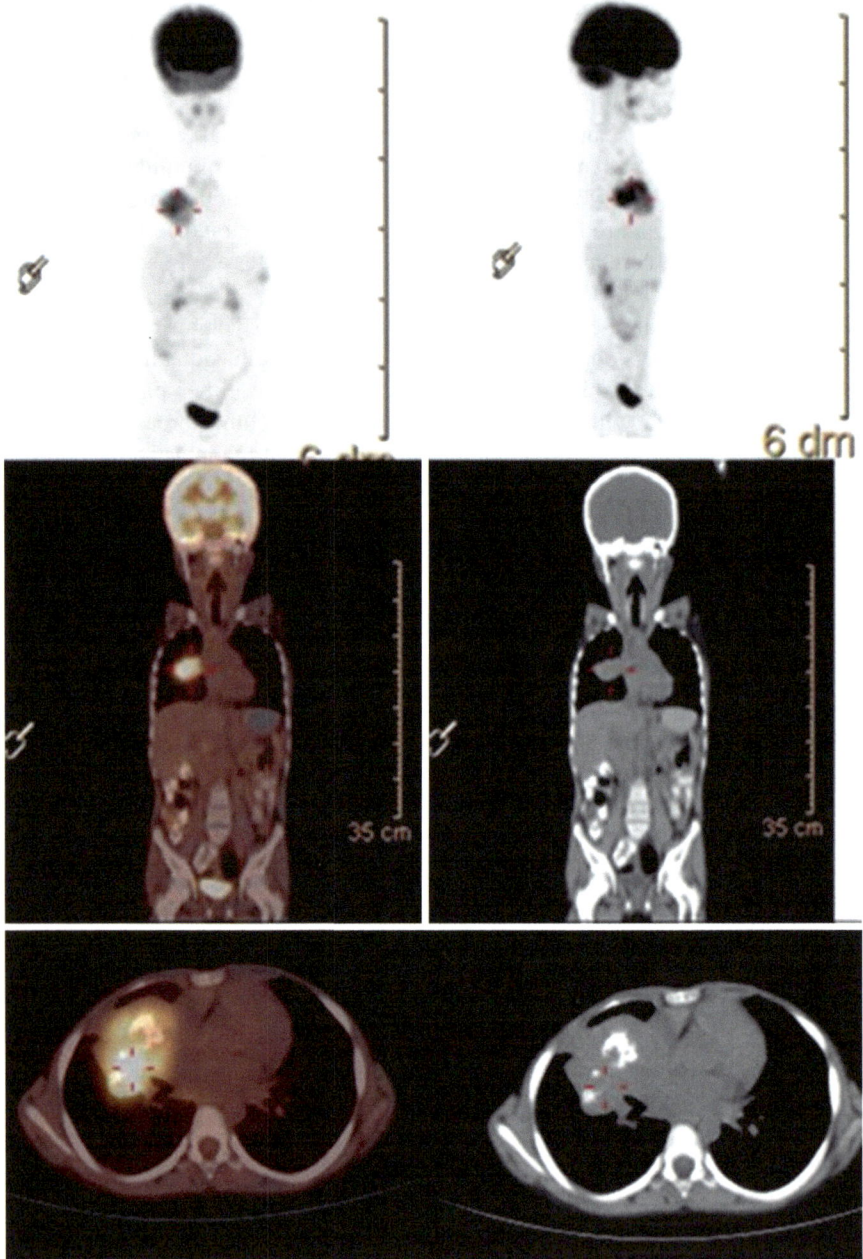

Fig. 9.3 Baseline PET/CT scans showing metabolically active lesion with calcification in right middle lobe in a patient of Inflammatory pseudotumor (IPT) of lung, a rare IgG$_4$ related disease entity (Reproduced with permission from Basu et al. [46])

Conclusion

Autoimmune disorders primarily cause inflammation in the target organ mediated by auto-antibodies. Since advent of PET/CT scanners, the applications of FDG in infection and inflammation imaging came to the fore. FDG PET/CT has demonstrated its potentials in systemic immune-related inflammatory disorders. Although most of the FDG PET/CT studies in imaging of autoimmune diseases have been undertaken in small number of patients and are retrospective, the promise of this hybrid imaging modality is obvious. With better planned prospective studies, FDG PET/CT has the potential to become front-runner in imaging and management algorithm of autoimmune disorders, especially for early non-invasive diagnosis and treatment response monitoring.

Key Points

- Early visualization of active inflammation caused by activated immune cells in the target organ is possible with FDG PET/CT, as against late tissue or organ destruction visualized by anatomical imaging.

- Compared to conventional nuclear medicine techniques, FDG PET/CT has high resolution and target-to-background ratio leading to better sensitivity.

- As autoimmune disorders may involve multiple sites in the body, whole body FDG PET/CT imaging is advantageous and can be undertaken in reasonably short time.

- FDG PET/CT can show the most accessible site for biopsy and help in diagnosis, where biopsy site is inaccessible.

- Individuals with autoimmune diseases have increased susceptibility for developing malignancy. FDG PET/CT can potentially image those malignancies in the same scan.

- FDG PET/CT with its ability to quantify metabolic activity at the site of inflammation makes serial monitoring of response to therapy possible.

References

1. Ramos-Casals M, Brito-Zeron P, Lopez-Soto A, Font J. Systemic autoimmune diseases in elderly patients: atypical presentation and association with neoplasia. Autoimmun Rev. 2004;3:376–82.
2. Kiss E, Kovacs L, Szodoray P. Malignancies in systemic lupus erythematosus. Autoimmun Rev. 2010;9:195–9.
3. Sela O, Shoenfeld Y. Cancer in autoimmune diseases. Semin Arthritis Rheum. 1988;18:77–87.

4. Bleeker-Rovers CP, Bredie SJ, van der Meer JW, Corstens FH, Oyen WJ. F-18-fluorodeoxyglucose positron emission tomography in diagnosis and follow-up of patients with different types of vasculitis. Neth J Med. 2003;61(10):323–9.
5. Zerizer I, Tan K, Khan S, Barwick T, Marzola MC, Rubello D, et al. Role of FDG-PET and PET/CT in the diagnosis and management of vasculitis. Eur J Radiol. 2010;73(3):504–9.
6. Basu S, Zhuang H, Torigian DA, Rosenbaum J, Chen W, Alavi A. Functional imaging of inflammatory diseases using nuclear medicine techniques. Semin Nucl Med. 2009;39(2):124–45.
7. Walter MA, Melzer RA, Schindler C, Muller-Brand J, Tyndall A, Nitzsche EU. The value of [18F]FDG-PET in the diagnosis of large-vessel vasculitis and the assessment of activity and extent of disease. Eur J Nucl Med Mol Imaging. 2005;32(6):674–81.
8. Treglia G, Mattoli MV, Leccisotti L, Ferraccioli G, Giordano A. Usefulness of whole-body fluorine-18-fluorodeoxyglucose positron emission tomography in patients with large-vessel vasculitis: a systematic review. Clin Rheumatol. 2011;30(10):1265–75.
9. Marienhagen J, Geissler A, Lang B. High resolution single photon emission computed tomography of the brain in Wegener's granulomatosis. J Rheumatol. 1996;23:1828–30.
10. Wildhagen K, Stoppe G, Meyer GJ, et al. [Imaging diagnosis of central nervous system involvement in panarteritisnodosa]. Z Rheumatol. 1989;48:323–5.
11. van Dam AP. Diagnosis and pathogenesis of CNS lupus. Rheumatol Int. 1991;11:1–11.
12. Bicik I, Bauerfeind P, Breitbach T, von Schulthess GK, Fried M. Inflammatory bowel disease activity measured by positron-emission tomography. Lancet. 1997;350(9073):262.
13. Neurath MF, Vehling D, Schunk K, Holtmann M, Brockmann H, Helisch A, et al. Noninvasive assessment of Crohn's disease activity: a comparison of 18F-fluorodeoxyglucose positron emission tomography, hydromagnetic resonance imaging, and granulocyte scintigraphy with labeled antibodies. Am J Gastroenterol. 2002;97(8):1978–85.
14. Treglia G, Quartuccio N, Sadeghi R, Farchione A, Caldarella C, Bertagna F, et al. Diagnostic performance of Fluorine-18-Fluorodeoxyglucose positron emission tomography in patients with chronic inflammatory bowel disease: a systematic review and a meta-analysis. J Crohns Colitis. 2013;7(5):345–54.
15. Lenze F, Wessling J, Bremer J, Ullerich H, Spieker T, Weckesser M, et al. Detection and differentiation of inflammatory versus fibromatous Crohn's disease strictures: prospective comparison of 18F-FDG-PET/CT, MR-enteroclysis, and transabdominal ultrasound versus endoscopic/histologic evaluation. Inflamm Bowel Dis. 2012;18(12):2252–60.
16. Jacene HA, Ginsburg P, Kwon J, Nguyen GC, Montgomery EA, Bayless TM, et al. Prediction of the need for surgical intervention in obstructive Crohn's disease by 18F-FDG PET/CT. J Nucl Med. 2009;50(11):1751–9.
17. Spier BJ, Perlman SB, Jaskowiak CJ, Reichelderfer M. PET/CT in the evaluation of inflammatory bowel disease: studies in patients before and after treatment. Mol Imaging Biol. 2010;12(1):85–8.
18. Malham MHS, Nielse RG, Husby S, Høilund-Carlsen PF. PET/CT in the diagnosis of inflammatory bowel disease in pediatric patients: a review. Am J Nucl Med Mol Imaging. 2014;4(3):225–30.
19. Das CJ, Makharia GK, Kumar R, Kumar R, Tiwari RP, Sharma R, et al. PET/CT colonography: a novel non-invasive technique for assessment of extent and activity of ulcerative colitis. Eur J Nucl Med Mol Imaging. 2010;37(4):714–21.
20. Yun M, Kim W, Adam LE, Alnafisi N, Herman C, Alavi A. F-18 FDG uptake in a patient with psoriatic arthritis: imaging correlation with patient symptoms. Clin Nucl Med. 2001;26(8):692–3.
21. Takata T, Taniguchi Y, Ohnishi T, Kohsaki S, Nogami M, Nakajima H, et al. (18)FDG PET/CT is a powerful tool for detecting subclinical arthritis in patients with psoriatic arthritis and/or psoriasis vulgaris. J Dermatol Sci. 2011;64(2):144–7.
22. Carey K, Saboury B, Basu S, Brothers A, Ogdie A, Werner T, et al. Evolving role of FDG PET imaging in assessing joint disorders: a systematic review. Eur J Nucl Med Mol Imaging. 2011;38(10):1939–55.
23. Beckers C, Ribbens C, Andre B, Marcelis S, Kaye O, Mathy L, et al. Assessment of disease activity in rheumatoid arthritis with (18)F-FDG PET. J Nucl Med. 2004;45(6):956–64.

24. Roivainen A, Hautaniemi S, Mottonen T, Nuutila P, Oikonen V, Parkkola R, et al. Correlation of 18F-FDG PET/CT assessments with disease activity and markers of inflammation in patients with early rheumatoid arthritis following the initiation of combination therapy with triple oral antirheumatic drugs. Eur J Nucl Med Mol Imaging. 2013;40(3):403–10.
25. Okamura K, Yonemoto Y, Arisaka Y, Takeuchi K, Kobayashi T, Oriuchi N, et al. The assessment of biologic treatment in patients with rheumatoid arthritis using FDG-PET/CT. Rheumatology. 2012;51(8):1484–91.
26. Kumar NS, Shejul Y, Asopa R, Basu S. Quantitative metabolic volumetric product on 18Fluorine-2fluoro-2-deoxy-D-glucose-positron emission tomography/computed tomography in assessing treatment response to disease-modifying antirheumatic drugs in rheumatoid arthritis: multiparametric analysis integrating American College of Rheumatology/European League against rheumatism criteria. World J Nucl Med. 2017;16(4):293–302.
27. Vijayant V, Sarma M, Aurangabadkar H, Bichile L, Basu S. Potential of (18)F-FDG-PET as a valuable adjunct to clinical and response assessment in rheumatoid arthritis and seronegative spondyloarthropathies. World J Radiol. 2012;4(12):462–8.
28. Mehta NN, Yu Y, Saboury B, Foroughi N, Krishnamoorthy P, Raper A, et al. Systemic and vascular inflammation in patients with moderate to severe psoriasis as measured by [18F]-fluorodeoxyglucose positron emission tomography-computed tomography (FDG-PET/CT): a pilot study. Arch Dermatol. 2011;147(9):1031–9.
29. Rose S, Sheth NH, Baker JF, Ogdie A, Raper A, Saboury B, et al. A comparison of vascular inflammation in psoriasis, rheumatoid arthritis, and healthy subjects by FDG-PET/CT: a pilot study. Am J Cardiovasc Dis. 2013;3(4):273–8.
30. Basu S, Shejul Y. Regional lymph node hypermetabolism corresponding to the involved joints on FDG-PET in newly diagnosed patients of rheumatoid arthritis: observation and illustration in symmetrical and asymmetric joint involvement. Rheumatol Int. 2014;34(3):413–5.
31. Sarma M, Vijayant V, Basu S. (18)F-FDG-PET assessment of early treatment response of articular and extra-articular foci in newly diagnosed rheumatoid arthritis. Hell J Nucl Med. 2012;15(1):70–1.
32. Faria D, Copray S, Buchpiguel C, Dierckx R, de Vries E. PET imaging in multiple sclerosis. J Neuroimm Pharm. 2014;9(4):468–82.
33. Sørensen P, Jønsson A, Mathiesen H, Blinkenberg M, Andresen J, Hanson L, Ravnborg M. The relationship between MRI and PET changes and cognitive disturbances in MS. J Neurol Sci. 2006;245(1-2):99–102.
34. Bakshi R, Miletich R, Kinkel P, Emmet M, Kinkel W. High-resolution fluorodeoxyglucose positron emission tomography shows both global and regional cerebral hypometabolism in multiple sclerosis. J Neuroimaging. 1998;8(4):228–34.
35. Derache N, Marié R, Constans J, Defer G. Reduced thalamic and cerebellar rest metabolism in relapsing-remitting multiple sclerosis, a positron emission tomography study: correlations to lesion load. J Neurol Sci. 2006;245(1-2):103–9.
36. Mishina M, Senda M, Ohyama M, et al. Regional cerebral glucose metabolism associated with ataxic gait—an FDG-PET activation study in patients with olivopontocerebellar atrophy. Rinsho Shinkeigaku. 1995;35(11):1199–204.
37. Otsuka M, Ichiya Y, Kuwabara Y, Hosokawa S, et al. Striatal 18F-dopa uptake and brain glucose metabolism by PET in patients with syndrome of progressive ataxia. J Neurol Sci. 1994;124(2):198–203.
38. Fisher R, Patel N, Lai E, Schulz P. Two different 18F-FDG brain PET metabolic patterns in autoimmune limbic encephalitis. Clin Nucl Med. 2012;37:213–8.
39. Rey C, Koric L, Guedj E, et al. Striatal hypermetabolism in limbic encephalitis. J Neurol. 2012;259:1106–10.
40. Shih WJ, Ghesani N, Hongming Z, et al. F-18 FDG positron emission tomography demonstrates resolution of non-Hodgkin's lymphoma of the parotid gland in a patient with Sjogren's syndrome: before and after anti-CD20 antibody rituximab therapy. Clin Nucl Med. 2002;27:142–3.
41. Nakajo M, Jinnouchi S, Noguchi M, et al. FDG PET and PET/CT monitoring of autoimmune pancreatitis associated with extrapancreatic autoimmune disease. Clin Nucl Med. 2007;32:282–5.

42. Lee TY, Kim M-H, Park DH, et al. Utility of 18F-FDG PET/CT for differentiation of auto-immune pancreatitis with atypical pancreatic imaging findings from pancreatic cancer. AJR. 2009;193:343–8.
43. Chen YK, Chen YL, Cheng RH, et al. The significance of FDG uptake in bilateral thyroid glands. Nucl Med Commun. 2007;28(2):117–22.
44. Zhang J, Chen H, Ma Y, Xiao Y, Niu N, Lin W, Wang X, Liang Z, Zhang F, Li F, Zhang W, Zhu Z. Characterizing IgG4-related disease with ^{18}F-FDG PET/CT: a prospective cohort study. Eur J Nucl Med Mol Imaging. 2014;41(8):1624–34.
45. Martinez-Pimienta G, Noriega-Álvarez E, Simó-Perdigó M. Study of systemic disease IgG4. Usefulness of 2-[18F]-fluoro-2-deoxy-D-glucose -positron emission tomography/computed tomography for staging, selection of biopsy site, evaluation of treatment response and follow-up. Eur J Rheumatol. 2017;4(3):222–5.
46. Basu S, Utpat K, Joshi J. 18F-FDG PET/CT imaging features of IgG4-related pulmonary inflammatory pseudotumor at initial diagnosis and during early treatment monitoring. J Nucl Med Technol. 2016;44(3):207–9.

PET and Infection/Inflammation

10

Thomas Wagner

Contents

10.1 Takayasu Arteritis

- Clinical details:
  - A 40-year-old female. Known Takayasu arteritis with 3 vessel gut disease. Bilateral renal artery stenosis and left subclavian artery stenosis. New mass lesion around the abdominal arterial tree. On mycophenolate mofetil and prednisolone
- Legend:
  - Moderate diffuse uptake in the thickened wall of the aortic arch and left subclavian artery in keeping with active large vessel vasculitis.

T. Wagner

Department of Nuclear Medicine, Royal Free London NHS Foundation Trust, London, UK

e-mail: thomas.wagner@nhs.net

© Springer International Publishing AG, part of Springer Nature 2018

T. Wagner, S. Basu (eds.), *PET/CT in Infection and Inflammation*,

Clinicians' Guides to Radionuclide Hybrid Imaging,

https://doi.org/10.1007/978-3-319-90412-2_10

- Teaching points:
  - Diffuse smooth uptake in the wall of the large vessels is suggestive of large vessel vasculitis.
  - The aorta is very often involved.
  - CT, MRI, and FDG PET are complementary.
  - FDG PET is useful to assess areas of activity in previously treated patients.

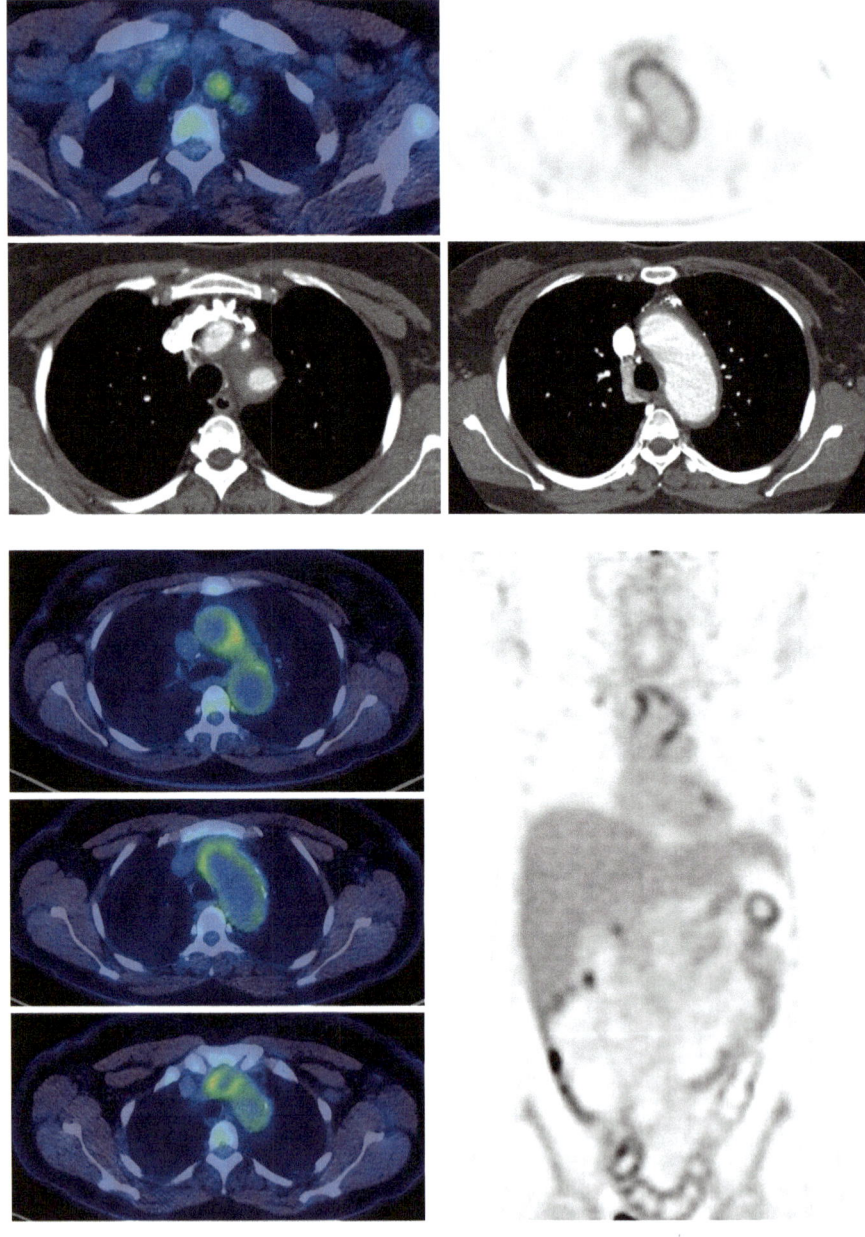

10.2   Giant Cell Arteritis

- Clinical details:
  - A 75-year-old female. Night sweats, anaemia, weight loss, and loss of appetite for a month. Raised inflammatory markers.
- Legend:
  - CT: mild thickening of aorta and great vessels consistent with aortitis
  - FDG PET/CT: Smooth linear uptake in the thoracic aorta, supra-aortic vessels, and abdominal aorta.
- Teaching points:
  - FDG PET/CT is useful the diagnosis of large vessel vasculitis.
  - Medium vessel vasculitis can be seen on PET/CT.
  - The role of FDG PET to assess response to treatment is not yet established.

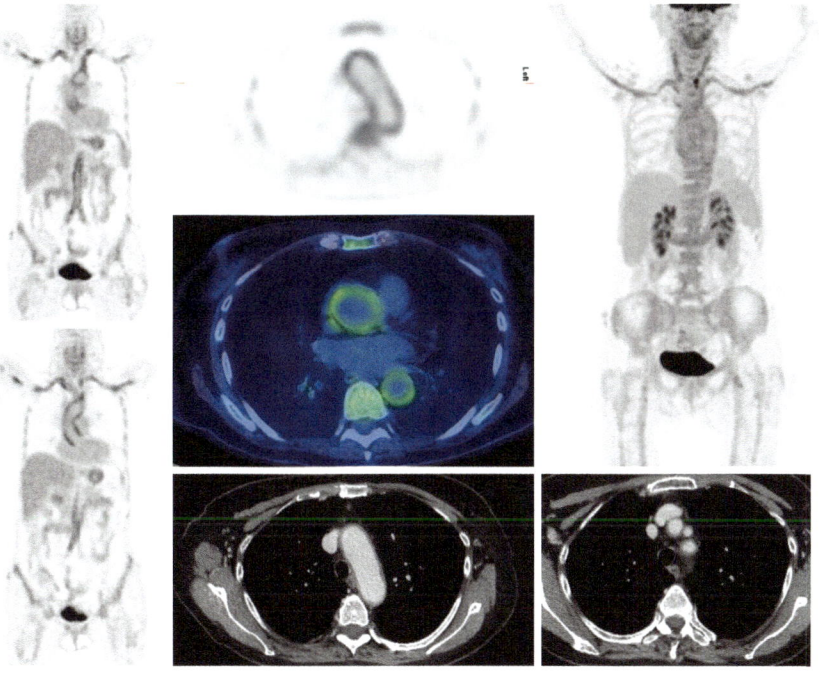

10.3   Psoas Abscess

- Clinical details:
  - A 60-year-old male. Previous medical history of aortobifemoral bypass. Raised inflammatory markers. Suspicion of infected graft.
- Legend:
  - FDG PET/CT: Intense uptake in a left psoas muscle abscess with adjacent involvement of lumbar vertebral body and abdominal aorta.
- Teaching points:
  - FDG PET/CT is useful to identify vascular graft infections.
  - FDG PET/CT can be used for assessment of response to therapy.
  - Normal non-infected vascular grafts often demonstrate diffuse moderate uptake.

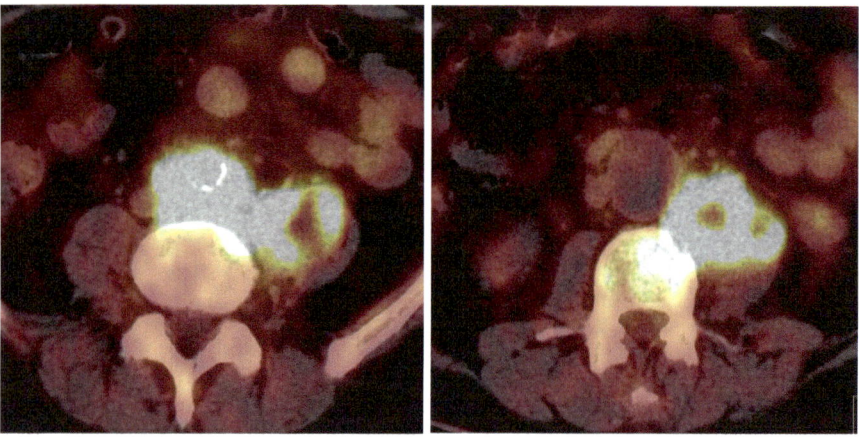

10.4   Infected Vascular Graft

- Clinical details:
  - A 80-year-old female with thoracic aortic graft
  - Suspicion of infection
- Legend:
  - Intense heterogeneous uptake in the aortic graft in keeping with infection. Diffuse moderate uptake in the cortex of the kidneys in keeping with amyloid deposition.

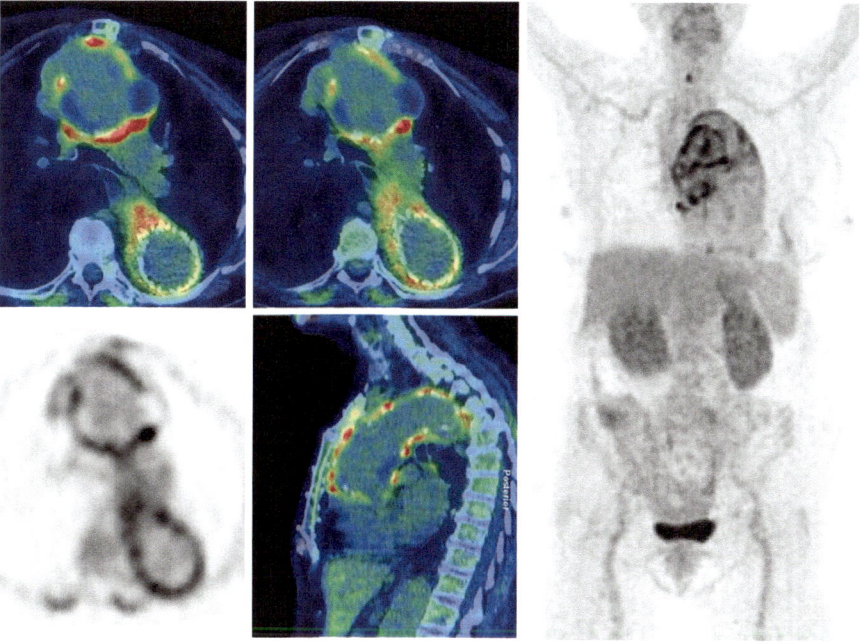

10.5   Infective Endocarditis

- Clinical details:
  - A 75-year-old male with infective endocarditis of mitral valve
- Legend:
  - Intense uptake in the mitral valve prosthesis
- Teaching points:
  - FDG PET/CT is not sensitive and should not be used for the detection of infective endocarditis of native valves.
  - FDG PET/CT is useful to detect septic emboli.

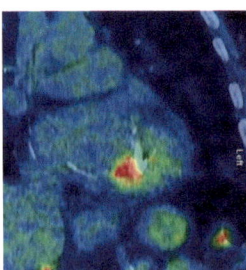 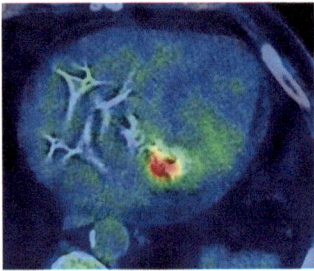 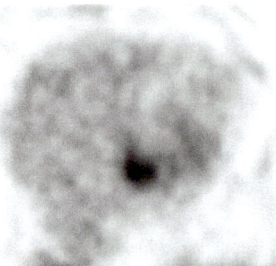

10.6   Pericarditis

- Clinical details:
  - A 55-year-old male with pericarditis.
- Legend:
  - Increased uptake in small volume pericardial effusion.
- Teaching points:
  - The level of uptake on FDG PET/CT will not differentiate between malignant, inflammatory, and infectious aetiologies of pericarditis.

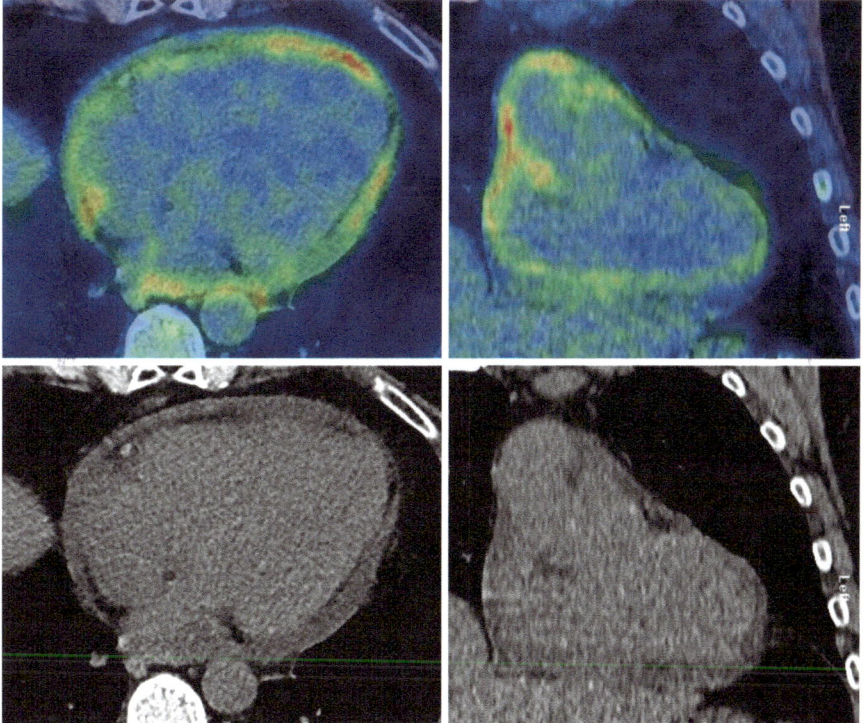

10.7   Peritoneal Tuberculosis

- Clinical details:
  - A 53-year-old male
  - Vague abdominal pain, nausea
  - CT shows diffuse peritoneal thickening
- Legend:
  - FDG PET/CT shows intense uptake in peritoneal thickening. No evidence of primary malignancy. Biopsy shows peritoneal tuberculosis.
- Teaching points:
  - Appearances of diffuse peritoneal involvement on FDG PET/CT can be due to peritoneal tuberculosis or malignant peritoneal disease.
  - FDG PET/CT is often useful to guide tissue biopsy to the most avid lesions.

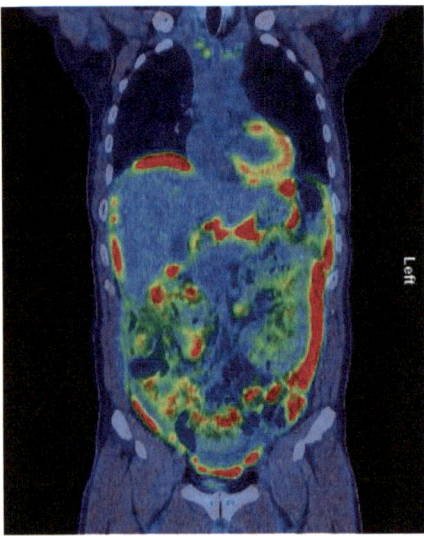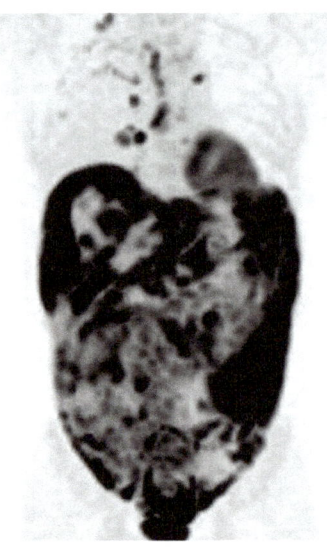

10.8   Skeletal Tuberculosis

- Clinical details:
  - A 43-year-old male
  - Swollen elbow joint, not resolving? tuberculosis, (all cultures negative) history of fever? any evidence of disseminated disease or lymphadenopathy
- Legend:
  - Intense uptake in erosions and destructive bone lesions in the elbow and the thoracic spine.
- Teaching points:
  - FDG PET/CT is highly sensitive to detect tuberculosis.
  - Tuberculosis, lymphoma, and sarcoidosis are three typical differential diagnoses that can have very similar appearances.

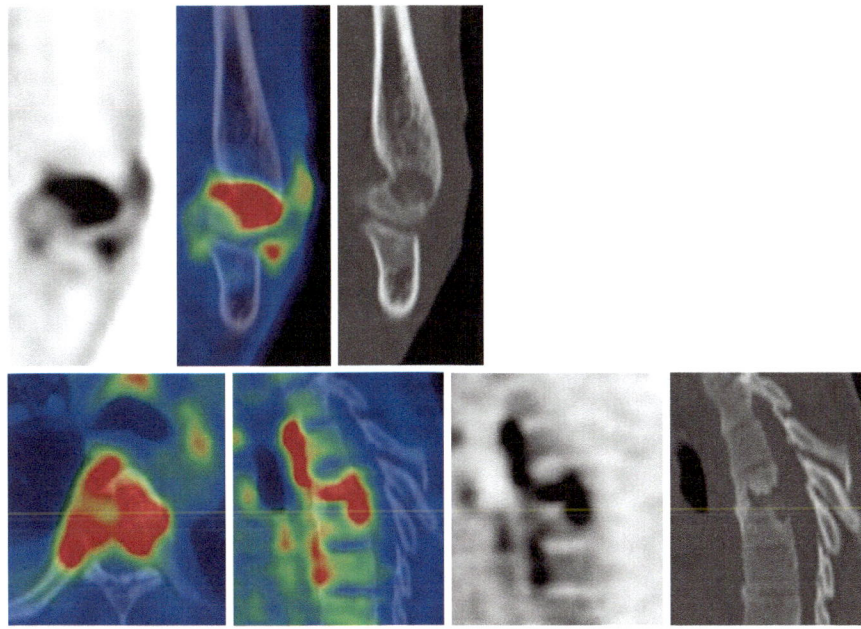

10.9 Spondylodiscitis

- Clinical details:
  - A 64-year-old male
  - Staph aureus infection
  - C6/7 spondylodiscitis
- Legend:
  - Intense uptake in a destructive lesion centred on C6/7 disc
- Teaching points:
  - FDG PET/CT is sensitive and specific for the diagnosis of spondylodiscitis.
  - It is often complementary to MRI.

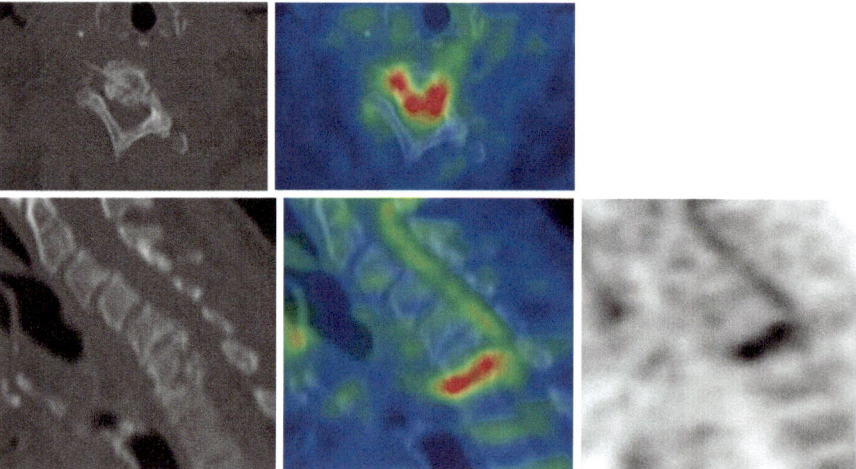

Index

© Springer International Publishing AG, part of Springer Nature 2018
T. Wagner, S. Basu (eds.), *PET/CT in Infection and Inflammation*,
Clinicians' Guides to Radionuclide Hybrid Imaging,
https://doi.org/10.1007/978-3-319-90412-2